Effective Communication in Practice

A handbook for bodywork therapists

Jan Pye   Wendy Jago

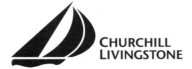

CHURCHILL
LIVINGSTONE

EDINBURGH LONDON NEW YORK PHILADELPHIA SAN FRANCISCO SYDNEY TORONTO 1998

CHURCHILL LIVINGSTONE
A Division of Harcourt Brace and Company Limited

Churchill Livingstone, Robert Stevenson House, 1-3 Baxter's Place, Leith Walk, Edinburgh EH1 3AF, UK

First published 1998

ISBN 0 443 05993 4

British Library Cataloguing in Publication Data
A catalogue record for this book is available from the British Library.

Library of Congress Cataloging in Publication Data
A catalog record for this book is available from the Library of Congress.

The
publisher's
policy is to use
**paper manufactured
from sustainable forests**

Produced by Addison Wesley Longman China Limited, Hong Kong
NPCC/01

Contents

Introduction

This book has grown out of years of practical experience with clients and in the training of therapists. It is based on our belief that with greater awareness and sharpened observation, therapists can learn to use the whole of the therapeutic encounter, not just the part involving their primary skill, to help the client achieve his or her goal. New therapists are understandably preoccupied with perfecting their primary skill and may sometimes overlook the fact that their treatment is a process that starts with the first telephone conversation, or initial face to face greeting, and continues throughout the primary interaction and beyond. They may also overlook, or indeed may not be aware of, the meaning that clients will be making of the encounter as a whole. This book is designed to help new therapists (and those in training) to extend their understanding and practical skills in all areas of 'communication' with their clients.

The first part of the book starts with who you are today. It is designed to help you to explore the various life experiences that have directly or indirectly shaped you. It helps you to develop a wider perspective on what influences the way you communicate, and hopefully more choices about how you can communicate in the future.

The second part of the book is organised around the stages of the encounter between client and therapist, and it works through each one. Our aim is to help you to make choices about quite simple, or apparently incidental, things which will make every aspect of your work fit with your wish to help the client and to help you to be as consistent as possible in conveying that message to your clients.

The third part addresses some important issues that arise when treating people, and offers some guidelines which may help. Again we are looking at effective and less effective interaction.

The fourth part is arguably the most important in the book – looking after the therapist! Effective client 'care' depends on effective therapist 'care' and covers such issues as supervision, avoiding undue stress and updating knowledge.

This book will provide you with an opportunity to reflect on all the component parts of the therapeutic exchange. We believe that it will help you to find ways in which your primary therapy can be enhanced into a rounded holistic encounter.

Acknowledgements

Many very special people helped to make this book possible. Our grateful thanks go to all of them, in particular our love to Leo, Charlotte and Terry for their support and encouragement.

PART

1

The therapist: knowing where you are coming from

The making of the therapist

Contents

1 The making of the therapist

Before looking at the skills of communication, we need to look at our own communications and our own personal style.

A wise friend, who had been a therapist for many years, once said to us: 'It is not the therapy which matters, but the therapist: that is why so many therapies are all effective.' What does this imply for us as therapists at different stages in our training and development? It means that the therapy has to be looked at as a series of interactions and interventions which are offered by one *person* to another *person* with the intention of helping.

This book is written primarily to help physical, i.e. body, therapists in training and in the early stages of qualified practice to recognise and have the ability to use every bit of their interaction with the client as a helping aid, not just those parts of the treatment encounter that involve their learned therapy.

From the very first moment that we are 'heard', maybe on an answerphone, maybe as we pick up the receiver in person, or perhaps through the written word in our reply to a letter of enquiry, therapeutic interaction can be taking place. Alternatively, in the worst case, those apparently routine or administrative parts of the encounter may be working against the aim of the therapy.

 Think for a moment about situations in which you have been the patient or the client. What made you feel, even from the beginning, that this person could, or possibly couldn't, be helpful to you?

Did you find their answerphone message friendly, or over-friendly? One message we heard began: 'Hi! This is Joe. What a shame you phoned while I was out. Try again later.' To us, it didn't feel very professional, and it didn't give us the feeling that he really cared whether we phoned back or not. Or what about the message that says: 'Sorry, folks, this is another one of those awful machines, but please do take the plunge and leave a message as I'd really like to hear from you.' A bit more difficult to assess? Yet we do assess these things – the language used, the tone of voice, as well as the content – in deciding whether this is the helper for us.

Move on a stage. If you have visited a therapist for treatment, what impressions did you get from their place of work? A clinic with a secretary and a waiting room: what kind of decoration? What sorts of magazines? Were there other people waiting in the waiting room with you? Were the chairs comfortable? Was coffee or tea available? Did the therapist keep to time? If not, what explanation, if any, was given for the delay? One hospital outpatients' department that we know now has a prominent notice saying: 'This clinic is running behind by … minutes today.' At least patients know where they stand.

What about a therapist who works at home? Lots more personal information to be gleaned here. We had one phone message, very apologetic, from a client's husband cancelling a first appointment. He explained that his wife had insisted he drive her past the house, and when she saw that the window frames needed painting (they did), she wasn't prepared to come. Sometimes the information gleaned doesn't reflect on the therapist's ability to do their therapy, as in this case; but in every case the client will take in a surprisingly extensive amount of information and make their own judgments upon it.

First, we need to go right back to the basics. Therapy is a series of interactions between two people, a patient or client with a particular issue or difficulty and a therapist with a set of skills that are relevant to that issue. When we first learn our therapeutic skills, we concentrate on the processes and the methods and their application to specific problems – if you like, the *content* of the *therapy*. Yet therapy takes place in a *context*, as we have been suggesting; it is in fact like the filling in a sandwich. But, as we all know, the total effect of the sandwich is achieved not just by the filling but also by the relationship between it and its outer layers: a roll can be soft, hard, crunchy; a baguette?; bread – is it white, brown or granary?; and so on.

Our message is not that one kind of outer layer is 'right', though some may be much less effective than others, but that *it makes a difference to the client*. Since we as therapists have the responsibility of organising the therapeutic encounter, at least initially, and of managing it even where the relationship is democratic and 'equal' in personal terms, we have many choices to make provided that we are aware of them, and we need to be aware of our *outer layers*.

This book is about those choices, and our intention is to leave you, as a committed therapist, with more choices at the end of the book than you had at the beginning. We believe, along with the NLP therapists John Bandler and Richard Grinder, that this is the aim of all therapy. In attempting to explore these choices, we are reminded of how we learned of their existence – not just in training but from our patients and clients. Even before that, we learned about many of them through our individual life experiences.

Therapy is *skill mediated through personal interaction*. So the therapist as a person is their major asset and resource. How do we become a person? Apart from our genetic make-up, it is through life experience. Our life experience gives us deliberate training (wait until you're spoken to; don't interrupt; stealing is wrong; give up your seat on the bus; never volunteer), but it also trains us through exactly the kinds of informal, involuntary and 'accidental' drawing of conclusions and observations that we have been talking about already. We learn from all kinds of things: the size of our family; where we came in the birth order of our brothers and sisters; illnesses and how they were dealt with; moving house or staying put; the character of our family members and friends; schooling; work and life events.

> We learn not only from major events and from what others intended to teach us, but also from our perception of these things.

Some businesses or helping agencies capitalise on this understanding and ask their employees to do a SWOT analysis: Strengths, Weaknesses, Opportunities, Threats. Some employers increasingly arrange for their workers to do a 'personal audit'. A nurse we know said that at the beginning of every training event she had been to, members had been asked to do a personal evaluation of this sort. It is rather like taking a personal inventory. You may have been asked to do this at some time on your training course. Even if it was not formally asked of you, you are very likely to have thought about yourself, your beliefs and feelings and how you arrived at them during the process of your new learning and through working with fellow students and teachers.

Since most therapies are learnt by mature students rather than by people straight out of school, training is often a major life decision in itself and may have been preceded by a lot of thought and self-analysis.

We would like you to look through the rest of this chapter carefully and to explore the topics and questions which you feel drawn to and to give thought to what that might be about. We are not asking you to work through the lot like a school textbook, but to shop around. Sometimes you may find yourself intrigued by something that hasn't previously occurred to you as significant; sometimes you may look again at something you have already thought a lot about. That is up to you. Like the rest of this book, this bit may be seen as a supermarket shelf with some goodies that you like or want now, and others which you may leave till later, or skip altogether.

We are not asking you to do something we haven't done ourselves. Although we have been in practice for a long time, our learning goes on. Writing this book is part of it, and we have asked ourselves a lot of questions about who we are, how we got here and where we are going. We expect that to continue. So not only have we thought up the areas and questions, we have also had a go at them too, and will give you some examples to illustrate what we mean from time to time.

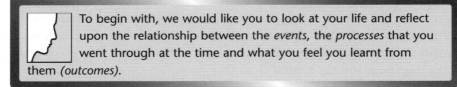

To begin with, we would like you to look at your life and reflect upon the relationship between the *events*, the *processes* that you went through at the time and what you feel you learnt from them *(outcomes)*.

This is a loosely structured exercise, which doesn't make any value judgments. The SWOT analysis that we mentioned earlier requires the person to make value judgments about themselves. This may make the process harder, and it also misses out one very important possibility – that of learning about ourselves without having to defend our actions. An insightful client of ours once said: 'When I now think about my life, I realise I can learn something useful from every one of my experiences, however dreadful they were.' Thinking about experience without classifying it in positive or negative terms makes it easier for us to think in a really open way about what each experience taught us, and about a range of ways in which we might make that learning useful.

Making a layered inventory

First layer – our individual experience

We suggest you take three headings: EVENT, PROCESS, LEARNING.

Write down these three headings on a largish piece of paper. We ask you to *write* rather than just think through in your head so that you are able to add more as you work through the book, and as further ideas and reflections occur to you and your learning continues to develop. That way you have a benchmark, or a series of benchmarks, for your learning. (We can't change the events of the past, but we can often profoundly change the meaning that they have for us.)

◆ Under 'event', just write the minimum *fact(s)*.

◆ Under 'process', write what you think you *experienced*.

◆ Under 'learning', write what you *were aware of learning* from the event/ process at the time, and also (if different) what you have since recognised you may have learned from it.

You may well find that new effects or results occur as you write. Learning includes skills and information, of course, but it also includes life beliefs and attitudes, such as those of the client who learnt as a precept what his father had learnt as life learning from his time in the army – 'never volunteer'.

We hope that working through the first layer of the inventory may have shown you how even the small, apparently randomly recalled events have significance, both events we have known about for a long time and others that we have come upon only now as we think about them.

It is often very informative to ask of an event or piece of interaction: 'What would another person have made of that?' It is an axiom of NLP therapy and training that 'the meaning of a communication is the *message received'*, i.e. communication takes place in the mind of the receiver. *Not the message intended but the message actually conveyed.* Taking this on board really makes us look carefully at the possible implications others may have drawn from what we said and did, but as we do this we gain more, not less, choice in our future communication.

We have called this a layered inventory because it is rather like a layer-cake (or a multi-decker sandwich). In this case, though, the layers are different because they 'slice' the same material – our lives – in different degrees of detail and abstraction. The first layer moved from factual detail to patterns of belief, attitude and behaviour. The second layer, which we are just about to ask you to look at, is a kind of recap, inviting you to see if there are any aspects of your life which might usefully be considered but which you didn't think of the first time around because you were working from the headings of your own experience rather than from an analytical list.

Second layer – our social world

Look at the list of headings below and see if they prompt you to add to the inventory you have drawn up so far. Please take a little time with each, using the same categories – event, process, learning. There is no particular reason for the order in which we have listed the items.

◆ Family
- number of children
- birth order
- extended family
- family or parental beliefs
- parents
- grandparents
- social and family activities
- family patterns and hobbies

◆ Education
- type of school
- friendships
- good and bad learning
- levels of education
- learning about learning
- location of school
- academic experiences
- social and sporting experiences
- favoured/disliked subjects

◆ Friendships
- childhood
- parental
- adult

◆ Role models
- real: who and why?
- in story or history: who and why?

◆ Recurrent fantasies, dreams and fears

◆ Work experience
- required skills
- skills learned
- social context
- good bits and bad bits

◆ Health and illness
- acute episodes
- chronic illness (if any) or allergies
- illness in the family
- hospitalisations
- drugs

- ◆ Holidays and time off
- ◆ Hobbies
- ◆ Adventures, traumas and major incidents
- ◆ Books, films and imaginative life
- ◆ Creative experiences
- ◆ Body
- ◆ Gender, sex and sexual orientation
- ◆ Likes and dislikes.

This second trawl through your personal history will, we hope, have helped you to add more information and make more links than you did the first time around. We discovered in completing the second layer that experiences as an only child gave confidence in handling one-to-one relationships and in being alone; a second look highlighted friendships with other only children, working easily in small teams and finding working in small groups more congenial than in large groups.

How do you feel your learning has influenced the way you live and work?

Third layer – philosophies of life

We believe that looking at our life experience and learning helps us to recognise where we are coming from as professionals, what our strengths are and how some areas of our skill and understanding may be less fully developed than others. Taking this inventory can help us to pinpoint where we wish to learn more, or where we might need to be aware of our learnt limitations.

As a result of our experiences, we will have arrived at certain explicit and implicit beliefs about the world, people and ourselves. These too are an important part of what the client encounters. In our experience, it is helpful to try to identify these beliefs or attitudes, so that we can maximise the usefulness of those that others may find helpful, and learn to modify or minimise those which, though valid in terms of the way we learned them, may not be so helpful to others.

'No pain, no gain' – an oft-heard maxim, particularly among psychotherapists. It certainly can be a logical life lesson for many people who have had to struggle for health, success or stability. Yet if it is part of the therapist's belief structure, what implications might it have for the therapy they offer or what they expect to happen to their clients? Take a moment to consider and write down some of the possible effects (both enabling and limiting) such a belief might have.

We would like you to jot down as many statements as you can that represent your beliefs about people, the world and living. Some may be straight repetitions of things your parents or teachers (or others who were influential in your life) said to you. Others may be conclusions drawn from your own experience.

It may help to use the following as prompters for other beliefs which are less readily accessible:

◆ I admire people who...
◆ I can't stand people who...
◆ Men...
◆ Women...
◆ One always ought to...
◆ Never...
◆ Lame dogs...
◆ Always...
◆ I have a right to...
◆ A thing worth doing....

You will undoubtedly think of others (please tell us for the next edition!).

What did you learn about yourself when you thought about your beliefs? Did you learn anything that illuminated your choice to be a therapist – specifically, to be a body worker? Did you learn anything about your attitude towards those who may come for your help?

We expect that many of your discoveries will make you feel good about yourself. Some may surprise you. Some may make you feel uncomfortable. Therapists are people. They are not perfect. It is one of our beliefs that we need to be aware of our strengths and make the most of them; we need to cherish our idiosyncrasies because these make us interesting, fun and very unique; and we can have choices about the bits we don't like *provided we recognise them and are charitable towards them in ourselves*.

The American therapist Carl Rogers said that one of the most important things a therapist could do to help his clients was to accept them, because in accepting them, particularly the bits they found difficulty in accepting about themselves, he showed them that they could be acceptable *as a whole person* – and this in turn helped them to work on their limitations and move forward.

This book is not about doing therapy on ourselves, but in the process of discovering and accepting all that we are, we become freer to offer to clients that which will help them and to continue fruitfully with our own growth and development.

Now that you have started to become aware of the layers that influence your perception, you need to focus on the skills and strengths that you currently have, and with your new-found knowledge use them as your chief/preferred tools within your communication process. Even our limitations, if accepted, can bear unexpected fruit, for ourselves and our clients. A colleague pointed out to us that 'our problems are our growing edge' – they occupy the place where sensitivity and energy are often found. If ignored, these tender areas can cause problems.

It is also the case that our very strengths can in some circumstances work against us: being good with a chisel doesn't make the chisel the best tool for all tasks. Therefore, as well as recognising and taking proper pride in our strengths, we need to be aware of their possible limiting effect and to try as far as we can to make productive use of our full range of qualities and skills.

The more we understand the need to possess, use and add to a repertoire of skills (in the very broadest sense), the more confident, 'tuned in' and effective we become in all our various areas of communication.

 We suggest you try the following three-part exercise, working with as many personal items as you wish. We have given two examples for each statement to set you thinking.

1. Through my experience I have learnt to...
   - anticipate discomfort and avoid it through tact
   - be very adept at getting alongside people.

2. A major limitation of this is...
   - not saying what I truly mean and then finding things backfire on me
   - people don't see the real me, only a mirror image of themselves.

3. I could extend my skill/strength by...
   - examining whether I am really protecting their feelings or avoiding conflict (and why)
   - examining when 'fitting in' could be seen as avoidance and investigating whether I am trying to avoid being my real self with people (and why that might be).

We have argued in this chapter that, whatever the therapy, the essential core of what is offered to the client is the therapist: their personality, their experience, their learning, their manner. These make up the vehicle which carries their skills. Just as many therapies are holistic in the way they regard the client, we believe that we are inevitably holistic in the way we approach the client – and that knowing this offers us richer information and richer choices.

As with all things, the more we understand, the clearer we become about how that knowledge can be used creatively within our lives. We hope that you have found these exercises a useful learning process that will enable you to go on and be more confident in the unique resourcefulness of your experience, which is the basis of your communication with clients and others.

PART

2

The process of interaction: the therapist-client encounter

Contents

2 How do they find you?

For the majority of you reading this book, it is likely that, up until this moment, the whole of your energy has been geared to taking your course and passing your final exams. Now you have to start turning your attention to where are you going to practise and who are you going to treat. Having decided on the kind of clientele that you would like to work with, your next questions are: 'How will I find them and how will they find me?' You may already have ideas of your own and this is a good time to jot them down, perhaps adding to them as you read through the rest of this chapter.

This chapter will explore the various ways that you can build up your client base. The most obvious way for people to find you is through written advertisements – within magazines etc., articles or your own literature – or by word of mouth recommendation. (One of the more obvious ways for you to find clients is to make use of your previous professional experience, but more of that later.)

Written advertisements – the concept

Let us give some thought to the written advertisement. If you do choose to advertise, make sure that your advertisement is consistent with:

- who you are
- what you do
- your target population.

The final point – your target population – is an area to which we suggest you give careful thought. Who you wish to work with will determine where you place your advertisement, e.g. the type of journal or magazine that you choose. Experience has shown that a large percentage of newly qualified therapists are prepared to work with 'anybody', and this is not something that we would take issue with, as such an approach provides knowledge and variety of experience which will be invaluable to both you and your clients. It may be some time later that you make the decision to specialise, in which case that will be the time to give thought to your area of advertising.

Whether you choose to specialise or to work generally, where you advertise is going to be extremely important to you, in that it will dictate your target audience. An extremely important consideration in looking at where you advertise will be the amount of money that you have available. Advertising space in professional journals and magazines does not come cheaply and you need to be assured that you will be receiving value for money. There are various ways that you can do this. The first is to check the circulation figures of the publication in question. Another way could be to contact one of the advertisers and find out what their take-up rate has been.

A large proportion of therapists, when they qualify, join their professional associations and it is worth checking with them to see what kind of publications have been used for advertising by their membership in the past.

If you do decide to target a particular audience, do make sure that your advertisement 'fits' where they are. For example, if you want to work with business people, talk *their* professional language. If you want to work with medical personnel, demonstrate that you understand medical terminology and be clear about where your therapy fits within the medical setting. Whatever the audience you are targeting, do not make claims that you can't substantiate. Even if you believe that your therapy can treat 20 conditions, do not list them all or you could be seen as a therapist lacking in substance. Pick out the two or three key issues on which you would like to concentrate, and let your advertisement sell this.

Give clear thought as to why people should choose you. What is it about you or your therapy or your advertisement that means people will choose you as against other therapists? Work at knowing what is unique about you, your approach and your treatment; don't be afraid to say what is your unique selling point, e.g.:

◆ 'As an ex-nurse...'
◆ 'Additional experience in America...'
◆ 'With a background in...'
◆ 'Twenty years' experience in...'

One of the more obvious ways for you to find clients is to make use of all your previous professional experience.

Take some time to think about previous professional experience. Can you see any links between previous experiences and your chosen therapy? Consider, for example:

◆ *Business.* Ten years in a business environment could have left you with knowledge of particular types of organisations, management styles, cultures and pressures.

◆ *Teaching.* Previous employment as a P.E. teacher can provide an invaluable link to athletes – professional and recreational – teachers and young people.

Both the examples given carry their own particular types of physical and emotional strain.

One avenue of advertising that we suggest you be cautious about is 'corner shop' advertising. Ask yourself, does it provide the right kind of atmosphere and professionalism that your treatment deserves? For many years, complementary therapies have been struggling to come out of the Dark Ages of 'hocus pocus', to establish a professional and scientifically acceptable footing. Everything that you do has to promote the value and worth of your therapy.

Your own literature

This is an important juncture for you to think carefully about advertising to the public. Think instead about the shelf life of your advertisement. A leaflet could be a better way of getting both you and your therapy known. Also, it travels easily and is versatile. It can be given as a handout at talks, left in surgeries and posted out in response to enquiries. Obviously, whatever form of advertising you choose will need careful preparation. Put yourself in your client's shoes: what are the issues about the therapy that would influence you and make you interested in a treatment?

Another form of advertising – which is also a service – is the provision of gift vouchers for your therapy, and these can be supplied throughout the year. (They can also be offered to companies as a 'support service' for their employees).

Personal – face-to-face advertising

Another form of advertising is face to face. One suggestion is to begin with the people about whom you have some knowledge, i.e. previous work colleagues and organisations, hobby groups etc. They can provide you with credibility and confidence even if you are newly qualified. Your past experience is one of your greatest assets; making use of it, trading on it, means that you are not in a position of having to cold-sell to strangers. You will be working from a knowledge base where people knew you, respected you and probably had a great deal of admiration for your courage in setting out to achieve something that was important to you, i.e. your qualification. Those old networks provide a source of clients. People who knew you were in training need now to know that you have qualified; let them help spread the word for you.

Many new therapists prefer to provide a written advertisement, rather than involve themselves in face-to-face/self-advertising. They are concerned about 'getting it wrong' or being 'asked questions that they don't know the answers to'. It is often the reason why giving talks is a source of great terror to many therapists! What you need to hold in mind is that you have knowledge of your chosen therapy, you have the experience gained from being a student and working with the doubts and misgivings and concerns of fellow students, and, most of all, you carry the belief in what your therapy is able to achieve. It is the energy that flows from such a belief that most people will find exciting and stimulating. We can pretty well guarantee that their questions will be geared to wanting more information and more knowledge and not to tripping you up and making you look foolish.

Remember, the more you practise, the more there is to learn. There is no need to be afraid. If you are giving a talk – to a large or small group – and you're asked a question you don't know the answer to, you can say: 'That is a really interesting point'; 'That is something that I hadn't given thought to before. Thank you'; or 'What an interesting way of looking at that. Thank you. I will now go away and think about it from that perspective'.

You will gain more credibility by admitting that you either don't know or are not sure than by trying to bluff and bluster your way through. Not only will you lose credibility by such behaviour but you will also downgrade your therapy.

It is vital that you prepare thoroughly for any talks that you are asked to undertake. Remember that the objective of speaking before an audience is to achieve at least one of the following:

◆ to persuade
◆ to inform
◆ to impress or convince
◆ to entertain.

Don't lose sight of your objective as you prepare your ideas and notes and remember the old maxim:

Tell them what you are going to tell them.

Tell them.

Tell them what you told them.

If you are giving a short talk, i.e. time is short, the following format will be helpful:

◆ Brief introduction

◆ An example or incident to gain attention and get your point across

◆ The main point or purpose of the talk

◆ Benefits to audience – to follow your suggestions, use your therapy etc.

◆ Summarise.

If you are giving a long talk, the following format will assist:

◆ Introduction

◆ Example or incident to gain attention

◆ Main point of talk

◆ Slides, overheads, statistics etc. to support main idea

◆ Benefits or action needed

◆ Summarise.

Above all else, be yourself, and only use humour in your talks if it is something that comes naturally to you.

What will be important is that you impart a balance of knowledge and enthusiasm, which as far as possible provides for 'hands on' experience. (This experience can often be the start of word of mouth advertising.) You will also need to display clarity concerning language and thought.

In face-to-face advertising, start from a position of confidence.

Who I am and what I do + who I was and what I did = the sum of my life experience to date.

This is a good time for you to do the above sum, adding up your skills, roles, strengths, experiences etc. How could you use this information in advertising your therapy?

Other forms your face-to-face advertising could take are as follows:

◆ You could give talks to local groups, churches, institutions, rotary clubs etc.

◆ You could set up visits to establish links and liaisons with health centres, dentists, adult education centres, schools, colleges, social services and other practitioners.

◆ You could suggest to local radios and local newspapers that they come and interview you as a new service setting up in their area

◆ If you hear of anybody running a raffle or seeking 'gift sponsors', don't be afraid of offering at least one free treatment

◆ A somewhat more adventurous, and highly effective, form of advertising is the radio charity auction. Many local radio stations now run auctions – at least one per year – when they ask people to offer 'services' for auction. The sponsors of the services are then advertised on the radio. (What a lovely way to advertise – it combines both the elements of giving and receiving, and it's good fun.)

Word of mouth advertising is far more tenuous than any of the above forms and it can be taken out of your control if you are not careful. Word of mouth advertising can work for you or against you, depending on your professional behaviour and attitude 'off the pitch'. Most people, once they realise your profession, will be evaluating you and your therapy. It will be up to you what opinion they form. A few 'tips' to help are:

◆ Always be the best you can be

◆ Keep abreast of new knowledge and techniques

◆ Never be rude about another therapist in public

◆ Never be flippant about the work you do

◆ Remember that even when you are off duty people will still make judgments on the basis of what you say and do.

> In any form of advertising, trade on the fullness of who you are today. Your experience as a therapist is not limited to the time that you have been in training.
>
> *Remember, the world welcomes you for your uniqueness of spirit, it rejoices in who you are, and treasures the knowledge of all you are becoming.*

3 The first phone contact

Therapy begins before the client ever sees the therapist. Remembering this can help us to make our side of the interaction, from the very outset, as encouraging and helpful as we can.

The first parts of therapeutic change take place in the person needing help. There is, first, a recognition that something needs changing, that something is not right; second, a recognition that outside help is needed; third, a casting about to decide what kind of help or helper. Only after these stages does the potential client begin to reach out to the actual helper.

This is important, because it means that the foundation of therapeutic work is already done before ever the client contacts you. They have already made some kind of commitment, to themselves, to effecting a change. They have decided that enough is enough, and that getting better is possible. They will also be prepared to give up time (from work and other commitments) and, if seeking private therapy, will have committed themselves to some expenditure. This chapter looks at the first piece of 'live' interaction between therapist and client – the first phone contact – and examines how we can use it to lay a productive foundation for our work together.

We have all sought help at some time or other – from doctors and dentists, teachers, school nurses, bosses and colleagues, friends and family – even if we have never consulted a therapist as such. So we have personal knowledge of the processes we went through before we began to explain what was wrong and what help we thought we wanted.

Take a moment to remember some of your 'first contact' experiences.

So, the client is already committed. Some will be more committed than others. They will have different ideas of what help means – some will passively expect to be 'fixed' where others expect to take an active part in their own therapy. Some may have agreed to come at the insistence of others. For some, yours will be the first kind of help sought; others may already have done the rounds of alternative therapies. Nonetheless, the client is there with a readiness of some sort.

Knowing this, we need to ensure that everything we transmit to the client is, as far as possible, consistent in its message. Think about the message you want them to receive. It needs to contain some of the following implications:

◆ I am ready to help you

◆ My therapy is effective

◆ I believe you have what it takes to improve your condition

◆ I respect you.

Being human, we give out unintentional messages as well as intentional ones. This chapter looks at how the most likely form of initial contact, the first telephone call between client and therapist, can be handled so as to maximise the meanings we want to give, and so minimise unintentionally unhelpful or inconsistent messages.

However, there is also another important dimension to the first interaction. The client is an individual who has reached the decision to ask for our help through their own method of approaching things. They have assumptions, fears, hopes and expectations which lie behind their questions and comments.

Now, because we have all spent a lifetime interacting with others, we know a lot about implicit or covert meanings, but we don't always know what we know. And when we are new to a skill, some of what we do know may not be as much in our minds as our concerns about managing what is for us a relatively new role. In other words, the acquisition of a new set of skills often pushes other skills into the background. We concentrate on those things which are newest, and which therefore occupy us consciously, and this sometimes prevents us from acting with automatic or unconscious competence. As an example, we may be so concerned to tell a client on the phone all the things we think they need to know, or we may be so concerned with finding answers to their questions, that we become less aware of how we are answering or the possible meanings and reasons behind how and why they are asking. Yet in a conversation with a friend or family member, where we are not 'on duty', we are much more aware of the subtleties of what is said and not said, of voice tone and of the way of conversing.

This first phone contact contains:

◆ information-giving

◆ information-receiving

◆ exploration of 'fit' (personal and professional) between therapist and client

◆ initial agreement about elements of the contract to work.

In this chapter we will cover all these. We believe that the skills required to manage this interaction for maximum effectiveness are part of our learning from other contexts from the earliest years of our lives, and that although it may feel a little strange and unspontaneous to think about 'managing' the interaction as well as delivering the information and making the appointment, these skills in managing the process of the conversation can be drawn from existing experience and polished, so that our part of the therapy really does begin with the first contact.

The process of making contact

In fact, the first phone contact may not involve two people talking to each other at all. Most professionals have answerphones, so most clients first hear their therapist's voice in a recorded message. (Going further back, a client may first form some impression of you through advertising or a business card, both of which are discussed in Chs 2 and 11.)

The answerphone message

An answerphone is a godsend. It allows you to work without interruption when you are seeing people. If you work at home, it allows you to choose when to respond to clients, and so protects your personal life. If possible, get an answerphone that allows you to monitor calls, so you can choose whether to respond or to leave the call to a more convenient time. In the early days of practising from home, the number of calls won't be that great, but as your practice builds up, you could get lots and find them quite an intrusion into off-duty time. If you work from other premises, you will need an answerphone to take out-of-hours calls or calls that come when you are working.

What should the message say? It needs:

◆ a name

◆ your number

◆ some expression of regret for not being available

◆ an invitation to leave a message and/or a time to phone you again.

These things are the overt content of the message. There is also the message the client receives from your phrasing, your tone and your pacing.

> We suggest you write out a number of versions of your message and practise it in various ways. It needs to sound friendly but professional. This might mean that you rule out 'Hi!', even if that is what you would say face to face. What difference would it make if you say 'hullo' before saying your name? Is that more friendly than you want to be on the phone, or is that just informal enough?

Obviously, you are not available. How do you say this? Do you apologise? Do you imply that you are busy but in (this may be better than implying that the premises are unoccupied – potential burglars sometimes check)? Do you give a time for the client to phone back, or do you say that you will phone them back? In our experience, if you make your own appointments, phone back within 24 hours or people will have looked for another therapist.

You could have a set-aside time, like one therapist we know, for people to phone you. In this case, your message could say something like: 'I am available/generally available to take calls personally on ... days between ... and ... times.'

> Having worked out possible forms of wording, try recording them on tape. Play them back to yourself and see how differently various versions sound. Get your friends and/or family to act as guinea pigs. Ask them what impression they get of you from the various versions and why.

We have often been told by clients that they decided to see us because they liked how we sounded on the machine. Think about phone messages you have heard on other people's machines. Borrow what sounds good, avoid what you find off-putting. Check for unintentional double meanings. One of us once left a message saying 'you can get hold of me on...' before realising how it might sound!

The person-to-person conversation

As we said earlier, the conversation at an overt level consists of the exchange of information about the nature, content and terms of the therapy. The hoped-for outcome is an agreement to work together where both feel that this is what they want. The conversation, at a covert or implicit level, is about the 'fit' between therapist and client (in terms of a sense of personal compatibility as well as agreement about the aims and appropriateness of the therapy).

It is really important that you feel free to decide at this stage whether you want to work with this client or not.

The client knows that they are 'shopping around' when they phone the therapist. They may well say 'I'll think about it and phone you back' (if they say this, this often means that they will not phone back but don't like to say they have decided against seeing you). They have as much information from the call as you do. In other words, both of you have lots of information about each other from this piece of interaction, which gives each of you an impression of the other as people – just as you would if you met in a shop or at a party. It is our experience that if you feel uncomfortable about a potential client on the phone, there is some good reason, even if you can't put your finger on it at the time. The same, of course, is true for the client, but therapists don't seem to feel so free to decide against accepting a client as is the case the other way around.

It's obvious that no therapist should say, 'I don't like the impression you give me so I won't see you.' But if you have doubts, it's better in the long run to assume that there is some good reason and to find a way to put the client off which they will find understandable. You might say that you are really busy in the immediate future and that for this reason they would be better to approach someone else. If you feel they might need a different approach from your own (e.g. a firmer kind of person if you feel they are manipulative in their approach, or a softer therapist if you find yourself feeling impatient with their woes), recommend someone specific if you know someone. You are of course entitled not to work with someone of the opposite sex in a body therapy, especially if you work from home, and you could just say matter-of-factly that this is the case and recommend they find a same-sex therapist (nominate a colleague if you know of one).

It is important to bear in mind that the key aim when turning away a client is that the client does not feel personally rejected. So you may have to tell a kind untruth in order to preserve their dignity. Anyone would understand that a therapist was too busy to take on a new client (particularly since most clients, once they have decided they want help, want it sooner rather than later). Anyone would find it understandable that, in bodywork, therapists and clients might feel more comfortable working with someone of the same sex.

In telling these polite lies, you have to bear in mind that, even if your diary is empty and you do not mind working with someone of the opposite sex, it is damaging to you and the client if you begin work with someone you are uncomfortable with. If they boss you around, or are difficult, in that phone call, or if you get a 'creepy' or irritated feeling in those few minutes, be sure you are likely to experience this even more strongly over an hour, or weeks, or months. Once you have begun, it is much more difficult to terminate the work.

First impressions are not infallible, but they are important, and they are the result of very rapid processing of information that goes beyond the obvious content of the interaction. We know this from social and work encounters. We process from a very early age information which is incredibly complex, and we learn to draw meaning from voice tone, pausing, pacing, even pitch and vibration in the voice. Because we are not paying conscious and analytic attention to these elements, we often can't explain why we feel someone is angry or tense or hostile, but we know they are. Experienced therapists have mostly learned to trust these initial impressions, but when one begins to practise, it is harder to offset a doubtful feeling against the need to earn and the belief that people in need deserve our help. They do deserve help, but not necessarily ours. We do need to work, but not necessarily with them. There are more clients, and more therapists, out there. The right match is what matters.

The aims of the conversation

Let's look at the agenda of the conversation. Each party has their own. But the agenda has more than one level. There are open, or *overt*, aims, and there are implied or hidden or unconscious (*covert*) aims.

The client's aims

◆ Overt

- to find out the prices
- to ask about the relevance of the therapy to the problem
- how long are the sessions?
- how many will I need?
- special or particular questions (therapist's qualifications and experience)

◆ Covert

- do I like this therapist?
- is this therapy worth the expense?
- how does this person compare with others I have phoned?

These aims may influence what questions are asked, how much emphasis the client puts on particular questions and how long they keep you talking. Some clients know what they want to find out and ask methodically, while others 'feel their way'.

The therapist's aims

◆ Overt

- to answer the client's specific questions
- to get enough information to tell whether you can help
- what help has the client had in the past?
- to cover information that the client needs but may not ask for
- how did you hear about me?
- to make sure client knows what to expect
- to reach agreement if proceeding

◆ Covert

- to find out if you want to work with this client
- to firm up a contract to work
- to avoid a lengthy phone call
- to find out how committed the client is
- is there a hint of a hidden agenda?

Answer the client's questions

This seems fairly obvious, but what is the question behind the question? 'Do you work in the evenings/at weekends?' sounds straightforward, but may reveal that the client is unwilling to give the therapy (and/or themselves) priority, or that they want to find out that it can't happen.

Factual information needs to be given directly. Be clear and crisp about price, session length, days you work, etc. Clarity says to the client that this is how it is (i.e. your norm). You can always build in variations ('I charge X for people in work and Y for unwaged and children'), and you can, if you want, imply some readiness to negotiate by using the word 'normally' ('I normally work Monday to Thursday'). If a client then wants to ask for an appointment on a Friday, what they will have heard is that they will have to explain why this is important or necessary. If you have another commitment on Fridays, though, say 'I don't work on Fridays'.

Some clients will already be sure that your therapy is relevant to them. They may have been referred by someone else who has been to see you, or by another professional, or they may have read up about different types of treatment for their problem. Others, however, are less sure. They need a brief description of what your therapy involves and how it can help this condition.

> Jot down and then practise a brief summary which could tell an uninformed client a little about your therapy and the kinds of things it helps. If you know of a layman's account which they might find useful, you can give them the author and title and a likely local bookseller, or refer them to the library if you know there is a copy there.

If it sounds to you as if another therapy might be more relevant, ask the client if they have considered it. The right match of client to therapy and therapist is the overall aim of the conversation. If you are not sure either, you can suggest that they might find an initial consultation helpful and that one of its functions could be that you help them to explore different ways of helping their condition. Tell them that, in that case, you would refer them to some other therapy or therapist, and that the value of the consultation with you would be just that – to consult and obtain an informed referral. That is worth your time and their money.

Get enough information

You don't want a case history, but it can be helpful to find out if the client has seen anyone else before you; how long they have had the complaint; and whether it seems to have any triggering circumstances or feelings. Follow your instinct. If the client is being guarded or monosyllabic, ask if it is difficult for them to talk freely at the moment. Often they will gratefully say 'yes', and you can then offer them a range of information about what you do and what conditions you work with, couching any questions you may have in ways that they can answer with a simple 'yes' or 'no'. For example: 'Does your partner/ boss know you are coming?'; 'Is someone in the room with you?'; 'Is there a better time for me to phone you back?'

Cover unasked questions

Most people want to know how much, how often, and what the chances of success are. But sometimes anxiety or shyness can make them forget to ask. A frequently unasked, and important, question, is what happens if a client has to cancel at the last moment. The issues involved here are covered more fully later in the book, but try to make sure that the client knows everything that is important or that might lead to confusion or misunderstanding if unclear at this stage.

How did you hear about me?

This is a useful question to ask routinely either at this point or at the first interview, since it helps you to build up information about where your clients come from. It tells you how many come via referrals from other professionals, from doctors, from clients you have already helped, and from advertising. There is no point in continuing to spend a lot on advertising, for example, if you find it has not brought many clients!

What to expect

It is a good rule to remember that you may think something is obvious, but that not everyone else will share the same assumptions. For example, clients who have had private therapy, or seen doctors privately, may expect to receive a bill at the end of the month. If you want them to pay each session, it's worth telling them at the outset. They might expect that if they make an appointment it will commit them to a course of treatment. If you work on the basis that they are only committed to one session at a time, let them know (this will reassure some who may be tentative). If any special clothing is to be worn, or alternatively if you will need the client to remove articles of clothing, tell them at this stage what your procedures are.

Reach agreement

Both therapist and client hope that this conversation will help an enquiry turn into an agreement to work. If you and the client seem to be feeling positive about each other, you could start making verbal assumptions that they are coming, e.g. 'In our first session, you will be able to tell me in more detail about...'; 'When we start work together...'; and so on. Talking in this way helps the client to imagine themselves into what it will be like to be your client, and will help them to make the decision. If they are doubtful, it will also help them to realise that they don't feel quite sure yet, and they will find it easier to say, 'I think I need a little more time to think/to consult my partner/to save up.'

Content that needs to be covered

A summary of the content that needs to be covered by the end of this first contact is given below:

◆ Length of each session (specify if the first session is longer)

◆ What the treatment consists of (state whether the first session is a consultation, or in any way different)

◆ How booked up you are (waiting list?)

◆ Whether you work evenings/weekends

◆ Cost per session (any reductions for unwaged/children/pensioners/block bookings?)

◆ Likely number of sessions (you may be able to say, 'Most people come for X sessions' or 'I usually find that for your condition...')

◆ How effective the treatment is for their particular problem

◆ Your policy on cancellations (whether you charge, how much notice is required)

◆ Whether they will need to undress (how completely)

◆ Whether they are likely to feel tired afterwards (can they safely drive home?).

There are various ways in which you can make sure the client gets all the necessary information.

Produce a leaflet

A leaflet can be sent routinely to anyone who enquires; this may shorten your telephone conversations. You can include a map, which saves having to explain how to reach you, where to park, etc., and you might like to include a brief description of the therapy and some key information about yourself, your qualifications and your approach. It can sometimes be very effective to have a question and answer format covering the most commonly asked questions about your treatment.

However, the more you curtail the telephone conversation, the less interaction there will be between you and the client, and hence the less 'between-the-lines' information you and the client will glean from each other.

If you work in a clinic, you may not talk to the client at all prior to the first appointment, and although the same covert dialogue will be going on, it will be between the receptionist and the client. The client will not be able to form a prior impression of the therapist, and whatever impression the receptionist makes will not be passed on to the therapist unless it is in some way unusual. Having a leaflet that can be sent to clients will fill in some of the blanks about you, but it is difficult to substitute for the other half of the dialogue. (Chapter 10 discusses these and other pros and cons of working in different settings.)

Write a checklist

You can write a checklist for yourself.

 List all the essential items of information the conversation needs to cover.

Once you have your list, make sure it is in some convenient form by the phone when you ring clients or when you are available for them to ring you.

Develop a 'patter'

Certain phrases will help:

'I usually find that this sort of problem...'

'People often like to...'

'Generally, people seem to feel...'.

You can also say things like: *'Perhaps you could tell me in a sentence or two what kind of help you are looking for, so that I can be sure that I'm the right kind of person to provide it.'*

This has two covert messages:

◆ It tells the client to be brief ('a sentence or two').

◆ It implies that if you say you are able to help then you are indeed going to be ('be sure that I'm the right kind of person').

 Using the checklist you drew up, practise explaining the essential items until they come fluently (perhaps with a tape recorder or with a friend, a fellow student or a colleague).

Information given by the client

Factual

Clients will give both intentional and accidental information during the first phone call. If they make a booking, you might want to make some brief notes afterwards to cue you in when they first come to see you. They may mention relatives, work, where they live, age or previous treatment. Anything you remember helps them to feel less of a cipher, more of a real person, when they actually arrive – for example, if they mentioned where they live, you might ask them if they had an easy journey considering the distance, or whether they walked as it was a nice day. This is part of becoming a professional 'putter-at-ease', and you can imagine for yourself how it might make you feel more welcome if someone remembered (or had troubled to register) things you said on first contact.

Emotional

Indicators of emotion (apart from explicit reference) may include:

◆ pitch and tone of voice

◆ confidence or hesitation in speech

◆ quavering or sudden faltering

◆ rapidity or gabbling, indicative of anxiety or confusion

◆ lengthy pauses and/or slow delivery, indicative of depression, confusion or some kinds of medication.

Language

The words we use and the structures in which we deploy them are a clear indicator of education (in its broadest sense). Together with accent, they may give you information on place of upbringing, social class, intellectual fluency and social sophistication, all of which will help you to pitch your explanations and to make a better fit for the client. We have spent years learning how to make assumptions on the basis of speech. Bearing in mind that assumptions are not facts, nonetheless we can gather a lot from the way the enquirer speaks to us and manages the business of finding out about us and our work.

> Jot down your impressions of the client after the first phone call, and after the first session look again at what you wrote. How accurate were you? If you repeat this exercise with several clients, and then again from time to time as your practice continues, you will begin to find where your areas of greatest accuracy are, and where your impressions are less reliable.

Phraseology also tells us much. Consider, for example, the differences there might be between 'Can you tell me...' and 'I don't suppose that...'?

Bear in mind, too, that the client will be reading between the lines just as much as you are. In constructing and practising your patter, try to use clear, simple, non-technical language. If it becomes obvious in the conversation that the client has some knowledge or previous understanding of your therapy, or a more complex level of intellectual functioning than you had expected, you can change the way you talk to match: 'It sounds like you have some experience of osteopathy, so you'll know how cranial work can...'; 'Yes, aromatherapy can influence emotional conditions quite profoundly at times because of the direct way the molecules of the oil pass into the bloodstream through the mucous membranes of the nose...'; 'Well, we're not entirely sure of the physiology of this process, but clinical experience has clearly shown that...'.

The attitude of the client to the therapist and the therapy

During this two-way exchange, we as therapists are forming an impression of the client's needs, background, education, sex, age, expectations, previous knowledge etc. Among our covert aims is to decide whether to work with the client, which includes assessing what their attitude is towards us and the therapy we offer.

When any of us converses with someone we perceive as an expert, we can't avoid giving some indication of our attitudes and feelings about experts and authority figures. There are no right and wrong attitudes, but because all therapists are individuals, each will find it easier to work with some people than with others, and each will find some expectations easier to meet than others.

Let's look at some possible hidden agendas clients may have, and how this may be revealed in the first contact.

Reassurance-seeking clients

Many people come with anxiety about their condition, and look to the therapist for reassurance: 'Can you help?'; 'Will it get better?'; 'Should I worry about...'; 'I've heard that...'. Try to be positive, but don't make categorical statements at this point as you don't have enough knowledge about this client and their individual condition. You can make 'usually' and 'generally' and 'often' statements, though it is worth bearing in mind that we are all inclined to hear what we expect, want or fear rather than what the person actually said. Feeling, in other words, has a strong and sometimes misleading influence on understanding!

Your training course will have emphasised that it is unwise – or even illegal – for you to assert that you can cure a condition. Understate rather than overstate. Make it clear that in your experience you have found that..., but that you will be able to provide a clearer idea of precisely how you can help the client when they have had time to tell you more at their first consultation. You might add that 50 people with the same condition are 50 different individuals, and therefore will all need to be approached differently.

Critical clients

Some clients come prepared to be critical. This may be because of their previous experiences with helpers for this condition, or because of their nature and their life experience. This attitude may be immediately apparent from the way they talk about doctors or previous therapists who have 'failed' them. Or it may be indicated more indirectly through nit-picking ('That seems rather a lot'; 'I thought you'd be prepared to work on Saturdays'; 'Well, of course I can't get off during the daytime'). They are unlikely to be direct, but instead may criticise other people or details of your treatment circumstances. You need to work with people who are prepared to work with you. It is not your job to change who they are or how they go about things (you are not a psychotherapist or counsellor, and they are not seeking that kind of help from you). If in doubt, or if you feel your hackles rising, avoid. Don't join in their criticism of others, but don't leap to defend others, your therapy or yourself.

Self-absorbed clients

Some clients are so self-centred that they have lost the awareness of what would be obvious to others, i.e. that this is a first enquiry of a busy professional, designed to establish the basis of a working relationship. They will be inclined to launch into a blow-by-blow account of the onset of their symptoms and may ignore your polite implication that an outline is all that is needed at this stage. Sometimes they even apologise for 'going on a bit' – and then go on a bit more! If you find you have taken more than about 10 minutes for the conversation and are having difficulty getting a word in, ask yourself how this might affect the therapy. Would this person tend to overrun appointment times, making it difficult for you to keep time for other clients? Might they pester you with out-of-hours phone calls? See how they respond to a firm indication that they are behaving inappropriately – 'I think that's rather more detail than I need at this stage'; or 'One more question, then I really have to phone some other people who also left messages.' In extreme cases, 'I think you're really getting into the kind of detail that needs to be saved for the consultation, so we should call a halt now.'

It is up to you as to whether you take on this kind of client or not. We all become more self-obsessed when we are ill or anxious, and when we come for treatment we have the right to the carer's full attention for the full allotted time. This first phone call, though, is a kind of 'freebie' which the therapist gives because they want to establish a working base – the time they invest now brings work and a living. But it should not be abused, and if you allow a client to override and overrun at this stage, you are setting a precedent for any future work you do together. Demanding clients are just that: some may want to work and to change; some may want attention and no change. If in doubt, or if you feel intimidated, pass them on to someone more experienced. High-maintenance clients, as one of our colleagues calls them, are neither 'good' nor 'bad', but not every therapist can work at their best with them, and it is harder to set boundaries when you are just beginning.

Arrogant and bullying clients

If a client competes with you, bullies you, name-drops or questions your competence and/or qualifications, avoid them. This attitude may not be obvious at first – perhaps all goes well until you begin to look for an appointment time. They may want to come early, or late, or they may quibble about fees, or tell you that you ought to be able to help in so many sessions (they have heard). Test your gut feeling by offering a really difficult time (very early in the morning, for example), or ask them to pay for a number of sessions in advance. If they willingly agree, perhaps your first assumption was wrong, and their apparent arrogance was a sign of something else (extreme nervousness?). If they resist, they are probably, at some level, resisting the therapy. Again, a more experienced therapist, or one rather different from you (or us!) might be prepared to take on this challenge. But why should you? The object is to set up successful therapy, i.e. for the benefit of both client and therapist. Don't take on what you feel is likely to be difficult or unpleasant.

'Professional clients'

People sometimes tell you that you are their last hope as they have seen everyone else. Tried the doctor, tried homoeopathy, tried reflexology, tried dietary therapy... This may be flattering, and of course we believe that our own therapy may well have something to offer that other therapies don't, *but* (1) what guarantee (or probability) is there that your therapy will be the one to work if all the others have failed?; and (2) could this just be someone who needs to keep a degree of illness, or to remain at the centre of professional attention for other reasons? In which case, before long they will be telling another professional how you in your turn failed them. This doesn't do you any good – it undermines your confidence, it may affect your reputation, and *it doesn't help the client either.* Avoid.

Dependent clients

Allowing for the fact that we all feel some diffidence when unwell and/or when seeking professional help, some people are more timorous and self-effacing than others. For many, you may be a means of building self-esteem and self-confidence. Working with them may involve urging/requiring them gradually to take responsibility for themselves through homework and other tasks as well as encouragement. On the phone, they may well sound diffident (perhaps with a hesitant manner and quiet voice). They may ask what you think and set you up to sound like an expert. It is not easy to tell them apart from clients whose dependency is a form of avoidance of taking responsibility, and who may phone you for emergency advice or leave frequent messages, driving you, your family or your receptionist wild. Often, the time of day at which the first message is left will be indicative. What kind of person phones a stranger's home at midnight? Maybe someone desperate – do they need the Samaritans? What if they want an appointment tomorrow? It could indicate a sudden emergency, or an unrealistic assumption that the world is out there waiting to fit around their needs. Check out these 'emergencies'. If the client seems self-dramatising, think hard about taking them on. One emergency may well be followed by others. If there is no hard evidence, but your sixth sense prickles, set some homework for them to do before the first appointment; for example, you could get them to write a brief history of their complaint, and log its variations daily for the intervening days. If the client then brings the homework in, they have shown a commitment and a readiness to work under your guidance and have done something genuinely useful which you can build on. If they 'forgot' or 'hadn't time', ask yourself what this may tell you about future work together. If necessary, you can make future sessions dependent upon completing assigned self-help tasks.

This may have seemed rather a dismal catalogue. But the same kind of information will also help you to distinguish from these initial conversations those clients whose need is desperate but whose courage is great; those whose intelligence or sweetness is going to make them a delight to work with; perhaps even those whom you will want to become friends with after therapy is finished. You will be calling on exactly the same kinds of evidence, but you will not need us to say 'go ahead'!

Dos and don'ts

We cannot see the client on the phone, nor they us; but as we have been arguing, there is plenty of information to guide both parties towards finding whether there can be a therapeutic match. Information is given both 'above the line' (overtly) and 'below the line' (covertly), but it is our job to try to ensure that our messages are consistent with our overall therapeutic intent and manner. This first contact sets the tone for what follows.

Availability and flexibility

If you are happy to be flexible in negotiating appointment times, by all means indicate it, but also be aware that some clients may take advantage.

If you feel comfortable with a degree of formality, indicate it by using the client's surname and your own: 'It's Mr Smith returning your call, Mrs Jones.' If you are happier to use first names both ways, use theirs ('Is that Janice?') and your name rather than your title ('It's Elizabeth Brown here').

Indirect messages you may give

◆ If you are busy, tired or upset, it is better leave the answerphone on as it will be difficult to concentrate fully on the client (the message communicated to the client by interruptions or impaired concentration is 'you are not as important as the rest of my life'). Answer, or phone them, at times that are convenient for you, when you are not rushing to meet a deadline (e.g. your favourite television programme starting in 5 minutes).If you must phone when time is limited, say so at the outset:

> *'I wanted to phone you today, so that you knew I'd got your message, but I only have a few minutes before going to a meeting. I can speak very briefly with you now, but I'd prefer to talk more freely: is there a time tomorrow when it would be convenient for me to phone you again?'*

It may be better to make this brief contact and arrange a later time to speak at more length, so that the client at least knows that you got their message and were concerned to respond to them.

◆ If you work at home, is it easy for clients to get through to you? If the evenings are filled with teenage conversations, this can cause you and your potential clients – and your children! – much frustration. Is it worth having another phone line just for your business (you can, after all, offset it against tax)?

◆ If your phone is answered personally, rather than by answerphone, ensure that whoever answers knows how to do it professionally. Clients shouldn't have to fight their way to you through small children 'being helpful'. And similarly, record any answerphone message at a time when there is no background noise – radios, TVs or even normal family chat in the background are all distractions from the professional focus you want to demonstrate.

◆ Reply speedily to clients' messages. A quick reply says you are attentive. A slow reply implies that you're not bothered, you're ill or you're away. If you are on holiday, your message needs to say that your practice is closed between X and Y dates, and to state whether you want clients to leave a message, consult a stand-in or phone back after a certain date. Some will wait (they have been told how good you are), others will need more urgent help.

◆ Speak with a smile in your voice. You want this client. You want to like working with them. You want them to like working with you. Be prepared to enjoy the conversation and your voice will say all these things.

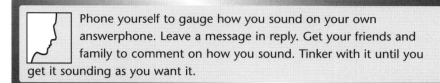

Phone yourself to gauge how you sound on your own answerphone. Leave a message in reply. Get your friends and family to comment on how you sound. Tinker with it until you get it sounding as you want it.

◆ Be available but not too available. If you say to a client, 'When would you like to come?', it tells them either that you are not busy or that they are in charge (of perhaps more than just the appointment time). If you have lots of free appointments, only offer a choice of two or three. This simplifies the choice and also allows the client to believe you are sought after. When you begin in practice, it also helps you to plan your diary (see Ch. 15) by bunching appointments rather than sprinkling them over several days and making it difficult to use your spare time productively. Better to have a full day and some empty ones than lots of bits and pieces. The client has, after all, made a decision to seek your help, and most will be prepared to fit in with your availability.

◆ Collect information about other therapists in your area so that you can refer clients where appropriate to other therapies, or, if you can't see someone as quickly as they want or if they don't feel right for you, so that you can refer them to another colleague within your own area of therapy. Have confidence that referring works both ways over time.

◆ Help the client keep the first appointment. Nothing is more annoying than someone not turning up for an appointment. To avoid this happening, you may:

– repeat the date and time arranged ('So we're agreed on Friday 22nd at 11, then')

– ask the client to confirm in writing that they are coming as arranged (particularly useful if the appointment is some time away, or after a gap such as a holiday)

– ask the client to pay for a first appointment in advance (with a confirming letter).

You can explain that the reason for these procedures is that you have now set that time aside for them, but that you do also have other clients needing help and do not want them to be turned away or to have to wait unnecessarily if for any reason this client is unable to attend as arranged.

Most clients, having once made the decision to seek help, will obey the 'rules' their therapist sets, if they can see that the rules make sense. At this point you can also tell them your policy about cancellations at short notice – again, the reason for asking for 1 or 2 days' notice of a change is so that you can offer the space to someone else in need. Even people wanting a cancellation may not be able to take it up if they only hear about it at a few hours' notice: they are deprived of your help, and you are deprived of income you could otherwise have earned. A full or partial fee for late cancellations (see Ch. 14) goes some way towards remedying this, and may also act as a deterrent – or, if you prefer, as a piece of preventative boundary keeping.

◆ Develop a clear set of instructions for how to reach your house/clinic. You might send a map, but if not, work out a clear set of local, easily observable landmarks by which to guide the client. Some will come by bus – find out about local bus routes and the names of the nearest stops.

> Practise giving directions to your workplace from different parts of town (and from out-of-town along major routes). Try them out on friends and family. Get them to tell you what you have left out, or what details are likely to be easily missed by a driver unfamiliar to the area.

Clients with cars will also need to know about parking. Some may be accompanied by partners, friends or parents. Where are these people going to wait? If you have no waiting area, warn the client in advance so that they can make plans (perhaps there is a local cafe or a library; or they may choose just to go shopping and return at the time you will be finishing). If you have a waiting area, let them know, and think about providing coffee/tea and perhaps a magazine or two to make them welcome while they wait.

◆ Don't accept a booking for someone else except in the case of young children. Often, enquiries are made by one person on behalf of another ('for my husband/my girlfriend/daughter'). Sometimes this is because the potential client can't easily phone (too public at work/too anxious/too young). Sometimes it is because the person phoning is trying to encourage or pressurise the potential client into coming. You don't know. It is important that the client 'owns' the therapy from the outset, so while you can discuss the therapy with the other person, ask them to ask the client to phone you at an agreed time for an opportunity to put questions directly, and to make their own appointment. In our experience, people whose appointments are made for them may not feel committed and may not even turn up. Without the direct person-to-person contact, both of you lack the sense of fit which this chapter has emphasised as being so essential to successful work. It could be there, of course, but it might not. You can explain this briefly to the person making the enquiry: it makes good sense, but in those cases where pressure is being put on the potential client it also conveys an indirect message that therapy only works if the client themself wants it.

◆ In the case of children, ask if the child themself wants help, or if they know why they need it. Find out what the child knows about you and your therapy. This is an opportunity to correct any misunderstandings about its nature and purpose, and to help the parent find ways to explain to the child what the therapy may be like. (For example, one child we knew asked at the end of a first session with a cranial osteopath when the treatment was going to begin!) Give the parent the kind of information you think the child will need, so that they come with some understanding of what will happen, and expecting that the experience will be safe and helpful. If you work at home, tell them what to expect ('We have a large but very friendly dog'; 'There is a toybox to play with while you are waiting'). All this helps to reassure the child so that they expect you to be friendly.

◆ Don't accept payment from third parties if you can help it. 'Owning' the therapy is one of the most essential components of its success. If someone else is paying, this may compromise the client's commitment, and often – especially in the case of an adult – takes away from their dignity. It also means that there is a shadow third party in the mechanics of the exchange between you and the client. This is particularly true with teenagers, or people who are dependent on partners, parents or friends (however kind and generous) to fund them. Ask the provider to give the client the money or the cheque so that the client can physically make the payment. This clarifies the exchange. If you explain your reason at the outset, most people can understand it, even if at first it seems a little odd. Again, be matter-of-fact ('my rule is...') and you will minimise any difficulties. It can also be useful to say in a very low-key way that, while you and the client appreciate that the parent/spouse etc. is paying, of course what goes on in the therapy is confidential between you and the client. This cleans up the interaction.

In this chapter we have looked at a number of features of what, at first, may seem like a very brief and practical prelude to the 'real' work of the therapy. Using our extensive, but often unrealised, skills at reading between the lines and hearing and saying more than just the words, we can get our therapeutic encounters off to as good a start as possible. We can set up the therapy in ways that give both parties the best opportunity to discover and agree a good fit before we ever meet in person.

4 Meeting and greeting

How you meet and greet clients will set the tone for the rest of the interaction and could influence the client's perception of the treatment. In this chapter we will look at preparing to receive clients, style and formality of greeting, and the need to be aware of what influences perception.

Preparation

First impressions do count and, despite what we may personally feel about this statement, it is worth taking this into account when you first meet a client.

Your client will be coming to see you because:

◆ they have been referred – 'They were so good, really helped me' (inference – therefore they could help you)

◆ they have been told about you and liked the sound of what they heard (inference – therapist was good)

◆ they have seen your advertisement – 'That looks/sounds good. I'll try it.'

Whichever route brought them to you, it is likely that their expectations will be high and, for some first time clients, possibly tinged with nervousness or anxiety. How you meet and greet your client will raise, lower or confirm those expectations.

Most importantly of all, be prepared for your client both practically and emotionally. Clearing papers from their chair as they walk in could say 'Sorry, I was caught up with things more important than you', or 'Sorry, I forgot you would be here so soon'.

It also means paying strict attention to time-keeping. Overrunning into the next appointment, and stating 'You don't mind waiting, do you?' subjects your clients to unnecessary and unwarranted decision-making and imposes on them a situation in which they may not feel free to object.

There may well be times when unforseen circumstances cause you to overrun, in which case it will be important that this is put to your client *along with the options open to them:*

> *'Due to unforseen circumstances with an earlier client, I am running approximately ... mins late, for which I do apologise. If you would like to wait, I will be with you just as soon as I can. If you are concerned that waiting might make you late for your next appointment, then I will be happy to schedule another appointment.'*

If you do agree to rearrange the appointment, you may want to consider the cost implications of your client's wasted journey and adjust your fee pro rata.

Running from one appointment into another could leave you with unfinished business from the previous client, which in turn could result in your being less attentive to your current client. We have all experienced talking to someone who 'isn't there', and didn't that make us feel just wonderful!

So preparation is the key. An aide memoire is invaluable and you can design one to fit your style. (Remember, pilots always go through their pre-flight checks no matter how many years experience they have!) Depending upon your particular therapy, such an aide memoire could cover such issues as:

◆ reception area and walkways (clinic), hallway (home) – clean and tidy, free of unwanted smells

◆ treatment room – affords privacy, clean, tidy, warm, well-ventilated

◆ previous client's notes – put away, i.e. not visible to current client

◆ robe, hangers and tissues available

◆ lavatory and hand basin clean; soap, clean towels, tissues available

◆ oils, powder, creams available for your own and your client's use (if appropriate)

◆ couch or treatment table clean and in position

◆ pen, consultation sheet (or last time's notes) to hand

◆ necessary reference books and diary to hand

◆ answerphone 'on' or telephone on silent ring/divert

◆ treatment music ready to play – if you use it

◆ other music turned off

◆ name of the client you are about to meet!

You may want to take a few minutes to add to this list anything that is pertinent to your therapy.

There will be an expectation – especially after the first telephone call – that you will be good and know your craft, so you will need to demonstrate this in your attitude and manner of greeting.

Give some thought to the new people you have met over the past months:
1. Who initiated the greeting and how was it carried out?
2. What influenced your response?

Dangers of stereotyping

Therapists need to be continually aware of the dangers of stereotyping. We talked in Chapter 1 of how beliefs and attitudes are formed by our experience of life, and in our interactions with our clients we need to be continually aware of the structures and filters that influence our actions. We all make judgments, and this is important to our day-to-day routines, but we continually need to ask ourselves whether we are making these judgements based on evidence and free of prejudice.

Look carefully at the following list. What does each mannerism convey to you, and what has influenced your attitude?

◆ Limp handshake

◆ Shrill voice

◆ Quiet speech

◆ Avoidance of eye contact

◆ Scowling

◆ Flippancy

It is probable that a great majority of readers will have had negative images. If this was the case for you in particular, please look again at the list and think about what else they might indicate. For example, a limp handshake could be indicative of a muscle-wasting disease or insecurity. Avoidance of eye contact could be acute shyness, embarrassment or insecurity.

It is important for us always to avoid jumping to conclusions, or making judgments, based on one indicator. We need to draw information and meaning from our encounters, but we should be wary of perceiving this information as absolute. We all have differing levels of self-worth, and this will affect our ability to interact with others.

Remaining sensitive and receptive

As we have already indicated, some of the new clients who come to you for treatment may still be a little unsure as to what is actually going to happen, and, in the case of osteopathy, chiropractic treatment, aromatherapy etc., how much clothing they will have to remove and how will they feel about the therapist.

Your initial greeting and your style of welcome should be designed to dispel some of their concerns. A warm smile of welcome, addressing them by name (always a good idea to use the name they gave you when booking their appointment), and a firm handshake convey that you are pleased to meet your client and always provide a good professional greeting. 'Hi, come along in' and a squeeze of the arm isn't quite the same and could convey totally the wrong image! Certainly, it might work for some clients, but not, we suggest, the majority. If this is your preferred mode of greeting, perhaps you might think about saving it until you know the client better and you are sure that it would be accepted in the spirit in which it was given. (We would flag here such issues as gender and cultural norms, and the need to be sensitive to such issues. Never presume, ask.)

Do not start any treatment discussions until your client is seated and you are also settled. The initial few minutes as you escort your client to the treatment room will tell you a good deal about how your client is feeling on many levels, and you want to be able to start processing this. Such processing does not mean fixing them with an unblinking stare, following their every movement and hanging onto their every word. Your overall aim is to assist, not give them a complex!

What we mean by processing is to allow your natural senses to work – to see, hear, sense and, in some cases, smell the person who is with you; in other words, to become aware of factors which ordinarily you might not give attention to, or might not take into account until later in the session. It is useful for you to be aware of how a client changes between the time they first arrive and later on in the session, when they have had time to compose themselves. It is also useful for you to be able to notice how your client might change over the period that you work with them, and to give some thought as to what might have caused the change. It may also be a useful piece of positive feedback for your client.

Some of the things that you might want to be aware of include the following:

◆ Are they quite early or late for their appointment?

◆ How do they return your greeting and handshake?

◆ How is their posture, skin tone and colour?

◆ What is happening to their rate of breathing?

◆ Are they full of chatter from the word go, or hesitant and unsure?

◆ Do they appear at ease or diffident and what gives you this impression?

(As discussed earlier in this chapter all are indicators, not absolutes.)

 There may be other things that you might like to be aware of. Take a moment to add them to the list for your future reference.

Some therapists may work in clinics where the receptionist is happy to escort clients to treatment rooms, or the culture of the practice may mean that clients find their own way to the therapist. Either way, we would suggest that as far as possible, new clients are greeted by you in the reception area and escorted to the treatment room. This will go a long way to building a relationship of trust and respect, as well as allowing you to start processing information.

Having escorted your client to your treatment room, do please indicate where you want them to sit. Many an embarrassing shuffle could have been avoided by such clarity. Give some thought as to whether you would like your clients to remove any garments before they sit down, e.g. coats, jackets, etc., and/or to giving them that option. As well as helping them to become more comfortable, it is also a useful way of easing them into the next part of the treatment process. This will be enhanced by your making sure that the client's first impression of you and your treatment room is the one that you want to convey – professional, knowledgeable and confident (see Ch. 11).

Think back to the first time you went to a therapist, dentist or new GP. What in particular do you remember that you liked? What, if anything, irritated you? Take heed!

In this chapter, we have laid emphasis on the importance of being prepared for your client, both practically – clean and organised treatment room, privacy, case notes to hand, etc. – and emotionally, e.g. being aware of the structures and beliefs that influence action and, in particular, the need to guard against stereotyping and jumping to conclusions.

Meeting and greeting the client is a time for being receptive to information and for settling and relaxing your client. It is also the benchmark by which clients can evaluate you and the rest of the treatment process.

5 The initial consultation

This chapter will explore the many functions of the initial consultation. From the therapist's point of view, it is about gathering information concerning medical, physical and emotional well-being, in a verbal and non-verbal way. It is also about making an assessment in terms of short-, medium- and long-term work.

From a client's point of view, he or she may require clarification of information already received – either from your initial telephone conversation or from paperwork you have sent. The most important thing they will probably require is knowledge of what is going to happen and how it is going to happen.

This chapter will therefore concentrate on information gathering and receiving, and the skills employed, the framing of questions and preparing your client for the 'hands on' part of the therapy.

We have stressed throughout this book that your therapy is a process and not an event. The process starts with the first time you and your client talk together about the proposed therapy. Each of the various segments of the therapy will take on different degrees of importance depending upon where your client is in their overall treatment process, i,e. whether they are at day 1 or day 21.

The initial consultation is, as its title suggests, the first consultation. Obviously the consultation process continues each time you and your client work together. The significance of the initial consultation is as follows:

◆ It will clarify the client's expectation of the therapy and any concerns or queries that you may have as a result of your initial contact.

◆ Most importantly, it will start the process of gathering the information that will inform the treatment.

◆ It will set the treatment plan.

In most cases, body therapists allow a longer first session in order to gather and give information. We have found that most therapists add between 20 and 30 minutes to the time taken to give a first treatment in order for this initial consultation to take place. In nearly all instances, this will be balanced with the need to provide a thorough first treatment. (If this feels rushed, learn from it and allow longer next time).

Initial sessions are often quite tiring for the therapist due to the intensive nature of the interaction and the volume and processing of information. So you may want to limit the amount of initial sessions that you do in any one day. If you are working in a clinic, you will need to remember to give this information to the receptionist in order that they can space your new clients and book in the required amount of time.

On a purely practical basis, it will be important for both you and your client to be comfortably seated for this part of the consultation. There is an ongoing debate about whether therapists should sit facing or to one side of their clients. We will leave this to your preference. We would point out, however, that if you are taking notes, you may find it physically easier to sit facing your client, thereby avoiding undue twisting and turning when writing your notes.

Another, perhaps more important, benefit of facing your client is that when you drop your head to write your notes, your client stays within your peripheral vision and thus you are able to note any changes in body posture that could occur when they think that they are not being observed.

Wherever you position yourself and your client, it will be important that you can each hear one another. Depending on the degree and personal nature of the questions asked, having to ask for something to be repeated does not lend itself to a feeling of relaxation and well-being. There is the added concern that you may record incorrect information.

We cannot stress enough the importance of talking your client through every stage of the therapy; this is particularly relevant for the initial consultation. (This process also gives the client the opportunity to clarify any issues left over from your initial telephone contact.) Some of the questions that you need answers to may not always seem relevant to your client, so, from the outset, explain thoroughly the purpose and function of the process that you and your client are about to engage in. Put simply, we suggest that you brief your client on the type of information that you are going to require, why you require it, how you will use it and, even more importantly, how you will store this personal information.

Before this process can start, you need to be clear about what issues the client is presenting (what is the problem) and what they are seeking from the treatment (what they want you to do for them).

Opening questions

As we stated in the previous chapter, (it is important that the clients have confidence in their therapist.) From the outset, therefore, we suggest that, having settled your client and assured yourself that they are comfortable, you ask the type of opening question that will set a context for the remainder of the therapy.

'So why are you here today?' is the type of question that requires the client to be clear about why they are sitting in front of the therapist; in other words: is there anything wrong; what are your symptoms? This could imply that some kind of negotiation will go on as to whether or not this particular therapist could be of assistance. A different question could be: 'How can I help?' This type of question could imply that the therapist believes that the client is very clear about what the issues are, and clear about what kind and manner of help they would require from the therapist. It also implies the therapist will be able to help.

It could also be argued that the first question is somewhat cold and slightly distancing, whereas the second question sets the tone for a two-way relationship. A third possible question is: 'So, what can I do for you?' On the surface this is a helpful and friendly question, but we would ask you to consider the 'do for you' part of the question.

Most body therapists today hold the belief that they are working *with* the client and that their therapy will become even more effective as and when the client accepts responsibility for their own life actions and behaviours. The phrase 'do for you' appears, at least on the surface, to be negating this principle and implying that the therapist will 'do it unto the client' and the client need not participate other than by being there. The counter argument to this is that the client is buying a service and therefore in asking that type of question the therapist is asking the client to be clear about exactly what type of assistance they want.

It has been our experience that some therapists feel that the nature of their therapy is both practical and physically orientated, but not geared to emotional intimacy. Such therapists may prefer the first form of exploratory question. Other therapists may wish to establish the bond that states 'I can assist you' and therefore ask a question along the lines of: 'How can I help you?'; 'How can I assist you?' etc. Others may feel that 'What can I do for you?' is a perfectly legitimate question to ask, as you have a skill which your clients are buying and in asking such a question you are also implying that you can fulfil that contract.

We do not feel that it is our business in writing this book to be prescriptive, but rather to raise awareness. It is not our intention within this chapter to explore the pros and cons of every exploratory opening question, but rather to raise awareness of your purpose in asking the quesion, what it is you intend to convey to your client by asking such a question, and what your client may infer from being asked the question.

Hearing and listening

Having asked your opening question, and having encouraged your client to explain their presenting issue, do make sure that you are hearing what your client is saying and not what you imagine them to be saying. It is a common failing amongst most of us that we often assume that we know what someone is talking about without actually checking back. For a therapist to regularly check back with their client that they have both heard the words used and understood the meaning not only implies good practice but also demonstrates that they are listening to their clients. Use such phrases as:

'Can I just check with you…?'

'Did I hear you say that…?'

'Let's see where we have got to…'

'Are you saying that…?'

Such phrases will indicate to the client your desire to understand and be clear about what they are saying. They will allow the client to recap, sometimes more succinctly, to clarify issues in their own mind, and possibly to give a new piece of information that provides an extra dimension. In turn, the therapist is provided with information that validates, contradicts or adds to what they originally possessed.

Another aid to hearing is to be able to cut out as much extraneous noise as possible, e.g. traffic and aircraft noise, noisy neighbours, music etc., and you will need to give this careful thought when you are choosing your treatment room.

Whatever the information gained, it is an important part of the process for the therapist to listen to the client without interpreting and, as far as possible, without interrupting, thereby beginning to understand the client's language and world. As Dr Richard Nelson Jones (founder executive committe member of the Britsh Association of Counselling) once said: 'It is very hard to listen when you are talking.' Newly qualified therapists, sometimes as a result of nervousness or lack of confidence in their skills, often fall into the trap of either asking too many questions or not giving their clients adequate time to reply. When asking questions, do give your client the time and emotional space to think, and do hear them out. They might not be answering your actual question, but they are providing you with information!

What does the client want?

It will be important for the therapist to be clear about what it is that the client wishes as a result of the treatment. Many clients, when asked to discuss treatment, will respond with phrases like: 'I want to be well again'; 'I want to be pain-free'; 'I don't want to feel so tired.'

What we immediately notice from such replies is that they tend to be negative. The client is telling us what they don't want and not what they do want. (Even 'I want to be well again' implies 'I don't want to feel as I do now'). You will undoubtedly find it very helpful when working with clients to help them to state positively what they require as a result of the treatment and also to explain to you what that actually means to them. For instance, 'I want to feel well' could carry the supplementary question, 'What does well mean to you?'. This kind of question immediately helps the client to visualise and feel their brand of well-being; they are already starting to imagine what being well will be like and therefore their thought processes and the work of the therapist will be moving in tandem.

Take a few seconds to think about replies you have given when you have been asked how you would like to feel, what you would like to do, what you hope to achieve, etc. Can you automatically answer positively about what you want, or do you find yourself answering initially what it is you don't want? What might this mean?

This is a very interesting exercise to carry out as so many of us are very clear about what we don't want, but less clear and less determined about what we do want. Think about questions or strategies that enabled you to move from what you didn't want to what you did want. Could you incorporate any of these into your work with your clients?

Taking a case history – the consultation sheet

Let us now spend some time looking at how you go through your initial consultation, i.e. how you collect the information. Research has shown us that nearly all bodywork therapists carry out their initial consultation via a consultation sheet. We referred earlier to seating positions when going through the consultation sheet and taking notes. Now we would like to concentrate on the framing and the placing of the questions. In other words, how do you ask your questions and in what order?

We are conscious that the uniqueness of the various therapies means that each will have their own important references. For example, chiropractors and osteopaths may place more emphasis on physical injury, accident, nature of current employment etc., while aromatherapists will want information on particular allergies, emotional issues, diet, etc. Throughout your training you will have used consultation sheets and become aware of the need for gathering concise, clear and accurate information. Your client will be able to assist you in this process if they understand why it is being carried out and how it will inform treatment. They will further assist you in giving concise information if you explain to them how long this part of the therapy is due to take. For example:

'What I would like to do now is spend the next 20 minutes gathering information about your medical history, lifestyle, employment etc. This information is important in that it will enable me to assess more clearly your current situation and the type of treatment I believe will assist you. If when we get to the end, you find you have remembered something important then please do tell me.'

Working through a consultation sheet demands the highest of skills from the therapist as they explore a range of issues from personal and emotional, to medical and lifestyle. They have to concentrate not only on the types of questions they ask, but also on the verbal and non-verbal answers they receive. (Body language and non-verbal signals and cues are discussed in more detail in Ch. 7.)

It is important for newly qualified therapists to feel comfortable with the layout and running order of their consultation sheet. The more comfortable and confident the therapist is in asking questions, the more relaxed the client will be, and therefore the more likely they are to provide the relevant information.

The client needs to be aware – as indeed do you – that all the questions asked have a direct relevance to the therapy. Why do you need to know how much your client weighs? Is it important that you know whether your client had chickenpox during their pre-school and early schooling years? Why is it important to know how many accidents, injuries and mishaps your 50-year-old client had during his school years? How would you define 'carrying heavy weights' when talking with people who have neck, back or arm problems? Does 'heavy' mean something that is too heavy for us to carry, or something that we have got used to carrying which is nonetheless heavy ? Please think carefully not just about why you are asking the questions but also about how you ask the questions, and in particular the use of emphasis. For example:

> *'How would you define* **heavy**?*'/'How would* **you** *define heavy?'*

> *'Are you* **comfortable** *with the amount that you drink?'/'Are you comfortable with the amount that* **you** *drink?'*

A difference in emphasis can imply a censorial or judgmental tone and probably not one that was intended by the therapist – we hope !

In many respects, human beings are very hard on themselves and are their own worst critic and judge. This often shows itself in glorious technicolour when they are asked questions about diet, stress, sleep, exercise, alcohol and smoking. Therapists therefore need to be sensitive to the fact that the slightest inclination in a judgmental way could fit with the client's own poor perception of themselves. This in turn could lead to their not being 100% truthful in some of their answers.

It is important that clients are constantly reassured, in both word and deed, that it is not the role of the therapist to make judgments about them or their lifestyle. Most certainly, if asked, they can provide assistance, guidance and knowledge, but they need to think carefully before telling a client that what they are doing is wrong. Therapists will often be given information which leads them to believe that what the client is doing is not necessarily in his or her best interest. A way of handling such information could be to say: 'You might find it helpful to…'; 'It might assist you if…'; or 'And if you did XYZ also, you might find that it's more beneficial'. Responding with phrases such as 'I don't think that's a very good idea', 'Why on earth would you want to do that?' or 'That's a crazy thing to do' is not the most helpful or reassuring way of handling issues.

Preparing the client for treatment

Having completed the initial consultation sheet and having clarified with your client the important information, you will now be starting to formulate the exact treatment. Prior to giving information about the type of treatment that you can provide, it might be useful at this juncture to reassure your client concerning the positive nature and outcome of your particular therapy: 'It has been found that…'; 'Experience has shown that…'. Such phrases help to move the client from possibly being caught up in their own particular experience to a knowledge that your therapy can assist in moving them on. As you go on to talk about the kind of treatment that you can provide for your client, it is important that once again you check back to make sure not only that they are hearing what you are saying, but also that they are in agreement with what you are saying:

'Does that sound alright to you?'

'Are you happy with things thus far?'

'Is there anything else you would like to know or ask about?'

This final phrase, in particular, provides the agreement to progress to the next stage.

The final stage for the initial consultation (and subsequent consultations) is the preparation for the move into the body therapy itself. And it is at this stage that you once again explain the practicalities of the therapy you are about to undertake. Initially, your clients will need to know the following. Do they need to move from the room they are in? How many articles of clothing do they need to remove? Where can they change and where can they hang their clothes? Do they wish to use the lavatory? It will also be useful for you to clear out any mythology: 'Contrary to what you may have heard, most people find that...'. Do run through the process before the start of the actual therapy: 'I shall ask you to.... then I am going to ...'. Then run through what they can expect as a result of the treatment: 'Some people find that...', 'You may experience...'. Clarify with the client: 'Is there anything else?' Try not to let them move into the next part of the therapy feeling rushed. And finally: 'Are you now comfortable and ready for the treatment?'

As we hope we have shown in this chapter, the purpose of the initial consultation is fourfold: it clarifies client expectations; resolves any queries the therapist may have arising from the initial telephone contact; starts the formal process of gathering information to inform treatment; and sets the treatment plan. Key to this process is the use of language, the framing of questions and active listening skills. We have used this chapter to illustrate 'good practice language' and lay emphasis on the importance of pacing your client and frequently checking back with them that you are hearing one another. To this end, the initial consultation should provide the therapist with all the necessary and relevant information – medical, family history etc. – to carry out a treatment, and should allow the client to feel reassured about the nature of the treatment, confident in the therapist's ability and the proposed treatment plan, and relaxed about the forthcoming treatment.

6 Involving the client in the process

Clients come with an in-built motivation – they want the therapy to work. So, at first sight, what need is there to 'involve' them? They have made a decision to come, made a phone call, arrived. Isn't this involvement enough?

In this chapter, we are going to look at what kinds of beliefs and attitudes drive the client, and how these may affect the progress and outcome of their therapy. We then consider how, through the subtle processes of 'ordinary' conversation, as well as through more overt motivating actions like tasks and home study, the therapist can encourage a more positive outcome through involving the client as an active partner in their own therapy.

Client motivation

Every client is different, and though most would avow that they have come to improve their condition, or in the case of relaxing therapies to spoil themselves or learn to relax, similar words may actually have quite different meanings.

What does 'getting better' mean?

For some, it means a complete absence of the symptom or condition that brought them to the therapist – rather like wiping out the recent past in which they have been suffering or have had their function impaired and just being how they were before. Some will even say this quite explicitly: 'I just want to feel how I did before I had this flu/before the car accident/before I put my back out.' They would like it to have been a bad dream, which fades away as the day progresses.

This may be realistic. The mind and body have a rare and helpful ability to forget pain once it passes, and many injuries and illnesses do leave little or no residue once healed. However, some clients will be finding it difficult to accept that their condition has some lasting consequences: the wearing away of osteoarthritic joints, the aches and pains of the ageing process, the problems of referred pain or the need to accommodate to permanent damage can all frighten, sadden and overwhelm clients. If the wish to return to a former state is unchanged, therapy is bound to be seen as a failure, at least in part. And although therapists need to encourage clients, and although in the majority of cases you will be able to offer the client real help, nonetheless you may help both them and yourself more if at the outset you help them to realise what is possible and what, in your view, is not.

This can be taxing. Many clients have already received negative messages, sometimes from other professionals, sometimes by making assumptions from other cases they have heard of personally or through the press. These can be just as unrealistic. There have been recorded cases of dramatic improvements from apparently fatal diseases when patients believed a new drug or treatment was going to provide a cure, and some equally dramatic relapses when further research 'proved' that the new cure was not quite as infallible as it at first seemed.

Clearly, a major factor here is the client's own beliefs and how these affect the body's responses to what help is offered. In responding to the anxious questions about how the therapy can help the client, we need both to be realistic about research or clinical evidence we do have (including our own experience with previous clients) and at the same time try to avoid giving them a deterministic view.

Choose a condition which you know to have a good prognosis for improvement, but which may involve some ups and downs that tend to discourage clients. Jot down a number of different ways of telling the client what they are likely to experience during treatment. If possible, get someone else to listen to you delivering each of these explanations, and to give you feedback on how they would feel and what they would expect if they were receiving them.

Now choose a condition which you know is very unlikely to change for the better, but which your therapy can help to manage or in some way alleviate on a maintenance basis. How would you explain to this client what you can do for them? As before, try various versions of your explanation and ask for feedback. In briefing your helper, ask them to listen to your tone of voice and to what is not said, but rather implied, as well as to the words you actually use. Watch out for prefacing words like 'unfortunately' or 'I'm afraid that...'. Words like 'generally', 'often' and 'usually' help to make the point that there are always exceptions (whether your expectations are favourable or unfavourable).

What kind of rate of improvement is the client to expect?

The client's view of what therapy may do for them often comes with a time frame, which may or may not be explicit. It is also closely linked with their beliefs about you as an expert helper. They may hope that treatment will 'fix' the problem there and then. Most clients visiting an osteopath may have some impression that osteopaths 'click' joints back into place. They will not necessarily know about tissue manipulation, or about cranial work, and they may not realise that once a joint is back in place, or realigned, inflammation can still take time to subside. Even the most gentle of body work can involve aching and tiredness afterwards. A tense client visiting an aromatherapist might feel wonderfully relaxed during and after treatment, but not understand how returning to a stress-producing way of life could quickly build up the tension again.

Clients who are desperate for help, who may have been the rounds of different therapies before coming to you, may well have acute – and sometimes conflicting – expectations. Their previous experience tells them that their problem has not responded to treatment (leading to a fearful belief that it may never respond), while at the same time they may hope that each new approach can offer them a miracle. Addressing these possibilities openly with them may be very helpful.

Practise some different ways of explaining to your client what they should expect from your therapy, immediately and as a result of several treatments. Relate the explanations to different conditions which you might commonly expect to treat. If you can't ask someone to listen and give you feedback, try putting your explanations on tape, leaving them for a day or two so that you gain a little distance from them, then listen pretending you are a client.

Think of visits you have made as a patient or client and explanations or predictions you have received. Try to remember what was actually said to you. What did you read between the lines? Was the overt message the same as the message you 'heard', or were they in some way different? What accounted for the difference? And how did the explanation relate to the eventual outcome of the treatment?

What has the client been told already?

If the client has already had help for their condition, they are very likely to have received some diagnosis or explanation before they see you, weighted by the expertise of the previous helper. Sometimes they will tell you what was said, but other times this may be forgotten as the two of you concentrate on building your relationship and exchanging relevant information. If you have an actual or mental checklist of questions to ask in your initial consultation, add some form of enquiry concerning what the client has been told. A colleague of ours pointed out how strongly influential such professional statements can be: the patient is often in pain or anxious and they are visiting an expert in the expectation of diagnosis or treatment. The mixture of distress, heightened awareness and deference to an expert means that anything they hear carries particular impact. In a very naturalistic way, the statement is hypnotic. It is heard by a mind prepared to be influenced, in a state of extreme concentration combined with dislocation from normal critical function. The diagnosis can become self-fulfilling because of the effect it has on the client, irrespective of how the problem might otherwise have progressed.

Do you know of any such statements? Parents, teachers and psychiatrists can all have this effect too. What was the statement/prediction and how do you think it influenced what happened/how the receiver felt?

How does the problem fit into the client's personal and family life?

The client is part of a network or system of relationships. In particular, they have important relationships with families and friends. Their physical difficulty does not exist in isolation, but in affecting them it also has an effect on the system within which they live. Like a pebble thrown into a pond, its ripples go beyond the point of impact, the sufferer, alone.

Acute, short-term problems make urgent demands on those around the sufferer. Broken bones or major strains may confine people to bed, or to the sofa, requiring others to carry more than their normal share of daily responsibilities. This disruption may make the sufferer extra keen to get back to normality – or it may give them a much-needed break from overwhelming but unvoiced pressure. Either way, there will be knock-on effects on their response to treatment.

If you find that the client improves then unexpectedly worsens, or if, conversely, they don't improve as much as you have every reason to expect, find out more about their personal system. One client whom we knew with irritable bowel syndrome had been treated by a variety of practitioners but her condition obstinately refused to improve. The most that could be done was to shift the pain from one location to another, though she was still spending a number of hours a day, in total, in the lavatory. Questions about her family system revealed that she lived with a disabled husband and daughter, each of whom needed her to perform various physical tasks that they could not do. Getting better would have meant that she would have had virtually no time for herself – their demands combined with her sense of obligation to them would have locked her into incessant to-ing and fro-ing in the home. The illness may have been stress-related in the first place; but certainly keeping it offered her some privacy, some reading and thinking time, even at considerable cost. It seemed that the problem needed to be unpleasant and unavoidable, because she would not otherwise have been able to be assertive enough to obtain any personal time and space. The unpleasantness also probably helped to divert both her and her family's awareness from the advantages which she did in fact gain from the condition.

Has the condition become part of the way the client sees themself?

Long-standing difficulties can become subtly integrated into the sufferer's self-image, and this can make it difficult for the sufferer to improve. You may notice a clue to this in the way the person describes their problem: 'I have to be careful how much walking I do because my back plays up.' The back has almost acquired an identity of its own. The person sees it as separate from the self, but this indicates both that they feel at the mercy of the offending part and that they also view it as a static or unchanging feature of their life (identity).

You can try commenting on this: 'It's interesting that you seem to think of it almost as if it were separate from you but ruling your life'. See how the client reacts. You might also ask about how they saw themself before the back became a feature in this way, which will remind them of a previous, normally functioning identity and which will imply that the role of the back in their life can change again. The sociologist Erving Goffman talks about 'spoiled identity' in his book *Stigma*, showing how people acquire and perpetuate such an impaired view of the self. Certainly if a person with a chronic condition is to improve, they are likely to need help in adjusting the way they see themselves and their condition. It is as though it has come into the foreground of their personal picture, and they need help in finding another, less prominent place for it. Even if the condition itself is only likely to improve to an extent, much may be done if they can lessen the extent to which it features in their self-concept. Labelling by experts is of course another way in which people's identity can become confused with their complaint.

Choosing motivated clients

If the client, as we have described, comes with beliefs and attitudes which can strongly influence the therapy, is there any way in which we can sort out from the beginning those who are most likely to benefit? In the chapter on the first telephone contact, we stressed how much information is available to us between the lines of an apparently ordinary conversation focused overtly on organisational and financial details. The innovative American psychotherapist Milton Erickson, when asked how he decided which clients to work with from among the hundreds who wanted his help, said simply: 'I choose those who are prepared to work'.

If you make it clear from the outset that your therapy may involve the client carrying out self-help tasks and exercises, or imply that you will be helping them change factors in their lifestyle which may be contributing to the cause or maintenance of their problem, you are likely to get some kind of response that will tell you how willing they are to do their part. Responses which imply that work/lifestyle cannot be changed may tell you that the client is unwilling to modify anything but expects you to do all the work. If you imply that people are often so close to their problems that they can't see the wood for the trees, and that part of your job is to help them find small manageable changes which can make a difference, some people will respond positively and with eagerness, while others reinforce their denial with more 'yes, buts'. Eric Berne in *Games People Play* identifies *Yes, But* as a 'life game', in other words a repeated unconscious strategy which involves listeners in sympathetic hearing about the problem, followed by suggestions of improvement. The 'yes, but' response tells the listener that it is sympathy not change that the speaker really desires.

Many clients, on the other hand, respond readily and cooperatively: 'Of course, I don't expect you to do all the work…'; 'Yes, I expected you would ask me to do some exercises/change my diet/take more rest', etc. Their quick understanding of the need to participate in their own self-management and healing is a good indicator of a working client – and a successful progress in therapy.

Because of our subtle and sophisticated between-the-lines understanding, clients will hear implications or presuppositions in the way you speak to them. Presuppositions like 'as we work to get you better…' or 'I usually allow 10 days between treatments so that you have time for some self-help tasks' tell the client in an indirect way what you are expecting. If the client then tells you that their work keeps them too busy to do any exercise(s), they have given you a clear message that they do not see therapy in the way you do. You may be able to help them change that, but you could, like Erickson, decide that this is not the client for you.

The role of payment in the therapy

If your practice is a private one, clients will be having to find money for your fee. This is a powerful motivator – though it can also result in the expectation that because you are being paid (such a lot – implied) you had better work for it. For the most part, however, cost is an involving factor, and helps to impel the client to get the most out of the therapy and feel they own it. We talked earlier about the value of token payments for just this reason, even if the person is receiving therapy at a discount.

Handing over payment at the end of a session is an enactment of the exchange which has taken place: it expresses the choice the client has made – to get better with your help – and the contract you have made between you to work together, as well as the recognition of your time and expertise. More dimensions of meaning, as well as mechanisms of management, are discussed in Chapter 14.

Agreeing a treatment plan

As we have shown, the initial session lays the foundation for the therapy. Explaining to the client what you plan to do and how you expect their condition to respond allows them to understand the process and to agree what the goals are. If you have said that your treatment only offers palliative care and this is understood and accepted, you have a clear, clean contract. If the client understands that what you do in the session needs complementing by self-help tasks, by self-medication or changes in lifestyle, and works on these things, you again have a clean contract with every chance of succeeding. Being explicit about what you plan to do respects the client as an equal, which in itself is involving because it treats them as a partner and not as an inferior. This may contrast very favourably with the way they have been treated previously by old-fashioned or arrogant practitioners or medical personnel.

One of us once asked a specialist treating her to explain technical language used in her presence between the specialist and another medical colleague, and was met with the response: 'I'm letting you listen, aren't I?' Put another way, treating a client as an intelligent adult encourages them to feel and behave like one!

The use of homework and tasks

Most people when they visit a therapist have some expectation that they may be asked to do something. Doctors' visits train us to expect instructions – take the pills; take a week off; put your feet up; rub in the embrocation. The expectation is there. Often body therapy will lend itself to follow-up by the client: Alexander teachers will show clients how to lie straight on the floor, how to rise from a chair, how to create 'space' in their armpits and 'widen' their backs. Aromatherapists are likely to prescribe blends of oils for use in the bath, in inhalations or in creams. But even where the therapy does not essentially involve homework, it is worth asking yourself if there is anything the client can usefully do to help themselves between sessions. Where we are involved in our own self-help we feel and become more independent. We get accustomed to self-care. We also learn to tune in to ourselves.

It can be really helpful, in the light of this possible alienation from self-awareness, to make self-monitoring part of therapy. Diaries recording the fluctuations of a condition, and its responses to treatment, thus serve a number of purposes. The client becomes actively involved in their treatment; they can through observation help the therapist fine-tune that treatment and assess its effects; and they learn, or relearn, a habit of noticing and respecting their own responses.

Tasks can be formal or informal. If the intervals between sessions are lengthy, keeping a diary or journal helps the client to remember details which might be forgotten if they relied on memory. Some therapists have found it helpful to use a duplicate book to record home tasks – a copy for the client and one remaining in the book for the therapist to refer to (both dated). If you set home tasks, you need to be sure to ask if they have been done: the message communicated by not asking is effectively that you forgot the client and/or didn't care. A duplicate record is a simple way to remind both client and therapist. If you don't use one, record the task in your case record, and check before the next visit.

Helpful tips for home tasks

◆ Make them simple, not complex, and ensure they are clearly related to the client's problem.

◆ Ask the client to perform the task only as often as you realistically think they will be able to manage. People have ordinary things to do and lives to lead. Even if you think it advisable to do the task daily, accept that every other day is probably the best they will manage: better a success with rather less than a failure at rather more.

◆ If you really want homework done every day, see if you can help the client to attach it to some regular and unmissable ritual already in their lives. Can it become part of a going-to-bed routine? Can it be done after (or before) breakfast or cleaning the teeth? Can it be done immediately upon returning from work? Pegging it to something which is already automatic will help to ensure it won't be forgotten.

◆ Check periodically that your tasks are realistic. Do you tend to expect too much? Are the tasks too complex? Do clients have time for them? Modify what you ask if you need to. Exhorting the client only gets you into a nagging-parent role and probably doesn't get the task done.

What if the client doesn't do the task?

In this eventuality, first ask the client why, and then check whether the reasons given indicate a design fault in the home task itself. This may allow you to agree a modified task which they will be able to do. Discussing the modification both reiterates the need for the task in some form and gives the client another chance to own the task as part of the therapy.

If the reasons are vague, or 'I just forgot', or if you get the impression of a lack of involvement or resistance, ask yourself: 'Does the client want to be passive in the therapy? If so, how do I feel about that?' Or: 'Is the client unconsciously trying to sabotage the therapy?'

Dealing with sabotage

First, work out what evidence leads you to think that sabotage may be occurring. Share with the client your impression that sabotage may be going on; give your evidence; suggest that this might be a reason for not doing home tasks/being late/ 'forgetting' appointments. How does the client respond?

We have talked about various reasons why a client might not progress, i.e. not believing that they can get better, having been told they will not get better, having to maintain their role as ill person in a social system. Are any of these operating in this case? Even if they genuinely want to get better, it is possible that other family members may have a vested interest in their remaining fragile, ill or dependent. Perhaps they invoke managing or caring roles which may suit partners or parents even if avowedly they too want the client to get better?

Sometimes it can be worth discussing this possibility with the client. For example:

'I just have a hunch that your husband rather likes to look after you. How would he feel, do you think, if you could go out walking on your own again? Might he feel that he had lost a role that he values?'

If you want to reinforce the client's belief that they can get better nonetheless (i.e. a way can be found), you could say instead: 'How will he feel when you can...?'

In some cases, clients whose progress is delayed or prevented because of emotional or interpersonal factors may need a different kind of help, e.g. psychotherapy or counselling or relationship work, and it will be to your professional credit, and very helpful to the client in the long run, if you suggest this. Always suggest that the reason for referral is because of the limitation of your skills, rather than implying that the client has too difficult or intractable a problem:

'I'm beginning to feel that you might benefit from an opportunity to talk these things through with someone who knows how to help couples in their relationships; and as that's going beyond my area of expertise I wonder if you would like me to give you the name of a colleague who works in this field, so that you and your partner can think about it together?'

Terminating therapy

If you feel the client is sabotaging therapy because they want to continue to fail, or because they want to prove you don't have the ability to help them (acting from poor self-image in the one case, and passive aggression in the other), you may have to consider whether you should terminate the therapy.

When we are relatively inexperienced, we are inclined to assume that failure to progress is probably our fault, and that if we knew more or tried something different, things would improve. By all means discuss the case with a more experienced colleague to get a cross-bearing on your impressions, but if you have done this and tried more than one approach, it may well be that failure to progress rests with the client and not with you. *It will do neither of you any good to continue if this is the case.*

Once you have decided that you should stop treating the client, bite the bullet and tell them politely but firmly that you feel you have reached the limits of your ability to help them and that the next session will be your last, one in which you will both have the opportunity to summarise what has been done and to say your goodbyes. Do not give, or accept, blame for this. It happens. Even if the client is sabotaging the therapy, they are not likely to be doing it malignly, but rather for complex internal reasons as much beyond their control as yours.

Once you have made up your mind, do not be persuaded to change it! No therapy could recover from this point. If you feel future therapy might be conditional upon some change, say so. For example, 'Once you have managed to sustain that exercise programme for 6 months on a regular basis, we might consider a few further sessions to consolidate the work and set an agenda for your self-care from then on.' This clearly implies that any further sessions will be conditional upon their actions in the meanwhile. Some clients, happily, will meet this challenge and return – in which case, you will be much happier to resume the work. Others will not contact you again and you will feel as if a weight has been lifted from your shoulders.

Static or stuck clients

Most therapists will at some time encounter a stuck client – one who may make some initial progress but who then fails to continue to improve. Sometimes this will be because the condition itself has reached a plateau. Sometimes it may be for psychological reasons. The therapist is unlikely to feel as irritated with this kind of client as with those who are sabotaging, who often provoke anger or dismay in their therapists. You are most likely to feel sad, or concerned, or even disappointed or a failure yourself. When you notice that a client's progress seems stuck, or when the client remarks on their failure to continue getting better, discuss the situation with them. It could perhaps be useful to continue to work with them on a support or maintenance basis, but it is important that this new contract is agreed between you. It is not helpful to continue to talk and work as if they were going to get better 'one day' if you think this unlikely. Better to say openly that it looks as if they have now reached a kind of plateau in their treatment, or that you think that this may be as far as they are going to get for a while, and to offer them a choice of what to do next.

There are various possibilities:

◆ to stop treatment altogether

◆ client to come at longer intervals for maintenance

◆ client to come at the same interval but with a support/relaxation agenda instead.

Bear in mind that, even if you feel you are not doing very much for a client, they may for their own reasons value continuing contact with you, and that this is a legitimate reason to continue if you also accept those reasons. One of us once asked a client whose progress seemed slow what she found valuable in coming, and her reply, after careful thought, was, 'Because this is the only place where I am listened to'.

Clients form trusting and important relationships with bodyworkers, and may well feel heard and cared for in important non-physical ways. For some people who lack close intimate relationships because of isolation, bereavement, age or lack of a partner, the importance of professional caring touch cannot be overemphasised. Discussing and agreeing a revised basis for the therapy allows the client to know that these reasons are also legitimate – they do not need to maintain a sore back or a painful bunion to justify continued caring and respectful therapy. Therapy which is 'stolen' through false pretexts is as hollow as a compliment that has been fished for – the receiver knows that the therapy, or the compliment, is partially invalidated by the means through which it has been obtained.

 Imagine a situation in which you might need to discuss terminating therapy, and practise different ways of telling the client.

Imagine how you would talk with a stuck client about changing the basis of the contract to continue therapy. Write down more than one version of how you would introduce the subject. Then check to make sure that you don't sound patronising. People who want to continue because of emotional rather than physical need are likely to be very sensitive to the implication that you may be sorry for them. Could they possibly read this into the way you have spoken?

The client comes with inbuilt motivation, and we need to be aware of the complex factors that influence what they expect and what they want from us. It is our belief that when the client feels they have an investment in their therapy, they are able to make fuller use of what it has to offer. Being aware of their possible hidden agenda can help us assess the meaning of their progress or lack of it, and can inform how we adjust our own behaviour and explanations to make them more effective.

From the very beginning of the therapist's contact with the client, natural and subtle means can be used to encourage the client's involvement as a partner in the process, to increase active partnership rather than passive dependence. Ongoing monitoring of the client's responses can lead us to an increased sensitivity towards barriers to improvement, and offers us choices as to what actions may be helpful for the client and for our own continued self-esteem.

7 ◆ The first 10 minutes

This chapter relates primarily to clients that you have seen at least once before. In other words, you have completed an initial consultation and given the client a treatment, and they have now returned for a second or subsequent appointment. Before any further treatment can be undertaken, it is important that the therapist engages with the client to understand:

◆ how they felt as a result of the treatment on the last occasion

◆ what has been happening to them in the intervening period

◆ how they are currently feeling

◆ how they would like to feel at the end of the treatment.

This last point is particularly important and we will come back to talk about it more fully as the chapter progresses.

Obviously the primary purpose of any body therapy is the hands-on work, but this cannot be undertaken unless you know what it is that is required of you: 'Before you set out, know where it is you want to go.' It is therefore vital that a brief period of time is set aside in order to discuss the issues highlighted above. For this to be effective and for the therapist to glean as much information as possible in the small amount of time available, he or she will need to be a skilled communicator. This means not only utilising their own verbal and non-verbal skills, but also being aware of the verbal and non-verbal cues coming from the client.

How therapists present themselves

We discussed in Chapter 5 the importance of seating arrangements in conducting the initial consultation and would emphasise that such seating arrangements are again vitally important for this part of the treatment.

Before we go on to discuss issues concerning your client, let us spend some time thinking about the best way for you to present yourself during this period of the treatment in order to encourage the client to relax and talk freely to you. The most important thing is to be sitting in a position where you feel comfortable and relaxed. You will need to decide for yourself whether it is important for you to take notes throughout this period or to make some brief notes at the end; this is something that is best left to your own discretion and that of the person you are working with.

Let us assume for the moment, however, that you have decided against taking notes. A comfortable position either facing or side-on to the client will allow you to observe their body posture and allow them to observe yours. What is important about your behaviour is that it encourages your client and that it does not distract them from their thinking. Therefore the more quietly you can sit and the less body movement you exhibit, the less likely you are to disturb your client's train of thought.

We are sure that many of you have worked with people who throw either themselves or their arms from side to side. If someone was exhibiting this 'windmill technique' whilst lecturing to a large group of people or working with a small group with a reasonable amount of space, then it may well go unnoticed or not be seen as distracting. In a one-to-one situation, however, where you are trying to establish a degree of professional intimacy, such movements can be not only distracting but also extremely annoying. We are not suggesting that you become a statue – which could be just as off-putting – but that you confine your body movements as far as feels comfortable to you. An upright position, hands gently folded or held on the lap, with feet on the floor or legs crossed, all denote professionalism.

Sitting in a yoga position because you find it the most comfortable is not necessarily the image the client would wish to see from their therapist. In confining your body movements, we are not suggesting that you shouldn't use your hands, but rather that you use them to emphasise a point and not necessarily to do the talking for you. To sum up, we suggest that you sit in a comfortable chair, one that allows you to sit upright without too much effort, with your arms in a comfortable position, displaying a posture that invites discussion. Sitting slumped in a chair, eyes to the floor, does not invite discussion!

It is also useful to think about how close you wish to place your chair to that of your client. This is not necessarily the time or the book to go into discussions about personal space but we would suggest that you bear this in mind when positioning the chairs. It will be important to both you and your client that you can change your body position, i.e. cross your legs, move forward in the chair, sit back in the chair etc., without impinging on the other person's space. At the same time it is important that if both of you sit back in your chairs, you can rest assured that not only will you hear your client but your client will be able to hear you. For your part you may be able to bridge this physical gap by raising your voice; your client, however, may not be in the position to do that.

When you are seeing your client for a second or subsequent appointment, and in order to assist the smooth transition from the first 10 minute slot to the primary therapy, it will help to give an indication of the time frame for this part of the session and the rest of the treatment process. For example:

> *'Let us just spend a few minutes checking up on what has been happening since last time so that...'*

> *'Before we begin today's treatment I would like to spend the next ten minutes talking about...'*

> *'Is there anything you would like to tell me before we start the body work? Let's think in terms of about ten minutes' discussion.'*

> *'As we discussed at the last session, my treatments start with a 10 minute recap on how you have been since we last met. Please tell me about what you have noticed.'*

You will find it a useful discipline and the clients will find it supportive to know what the whole treatment framework is. As Robert Frost once said, 'Good fences make good neighbours'. In other words, the clearer the framework, the more secure and relaxed the client feels, and therefore the more successful the treatment is likely to be.

Use of questions

We talked in Chapter 5 about the importance of opening questions and the hidden meanings that clients may feel are implied in the therapist's questions. An opening question could well be: 'So how are you this week?', 'How have things been since we last met?', or 'How did you feel after your last treatment?'. Any of these are warm and inviting questions. They are also known as open-ended questions, in other words they are open to your client giving you more information.

Examples of closed questions could be:

> *'So, have things been good for you since we last met?'*

> *'Have you felt better since the last treatment?'*

> *'Have your symptoms increased or decreased since we last met?'*

The difference between the open-ended question and the closed question is quite simply the type of response that you are asking your client to give. It will be important in your use of questions that you do not use them to guide your client down a particular route that you believe is either best for them or is the source of their problems. Your role is not to mind-read or second guess your client but to pace them and discover as much about them and their lifestyle as you can. Metaphorically speaking, you walk alongside your client, you do not lead them. As the purpose of this part of the treatment is to gain information to inform the hands-on treatment, it will be important not only that you ask the right kind of questions to elicit such information, but that you are also receptive to what you are being told. This means keeping yourself as open and as free of prejudice and judgment as you can possibly be.

Take a moment to think about 'stereotyping phrases' that are still in common use, e.g.

◆ black people are more athletic than white people

◆ gay men are more sensitive then straight men

◆ people who are overweight eat too much

◆ people who don't exercise don't care about their bodies.

As well as continuing to be aware of such stereotyping phrases, we also need to be alert to how they can influence our verbal responses, e.g.

'All single parents have it tough.'

A typical response could be, 'It must be difficult managing alone' (negative presupposition). A more effective response could be, 'So how do *you* find it?' (open question, no presuppositions).

 Look at the above stereotypes. Are these or others held by you? If so, take a moment to think about how they might affect your practice.

You will be aided in the process of 'being receptive' by having the fewest possible distractions in your treatment room. Therefore, being conscious of temperature, light and noise is going to be an important consideration.

As you start this initial part of the treatment, do remember once again to ensure that your answerphone is on and that the necessary windows and blinds are drawn to provide privacy, and that sunlight is not shining directly into either your client's or your own eyes.

It is going to be important in this session that you pace your client (move at their pace) and that you build on, expand and clarify what you are being told. In order to reach this clarification you will need to be using all your interpersonal skills as you will need to encourage the client to explore how they are feeling – without seeming to interrogate – and to make sense of this for themselves. Examples of useful introductory questions are:

'How have you felt since last time?'

'What was the most useful thing you took away from the treatment?'

'What short-term/long-term effects did you notice?'

'If I asked you to give a figure out of 10, how are you feeling today?'

You might then need to focus more sharply by asking questions that require the client to search for more specific answers, for example:

'Are you happy to tell me about...?'

'It seems to me that what you are saying is...'

'So the most important thing was...'

'So, overall...'

'Do you think it is connected with...?'

'So it seems to you as if...'

Active listening

A key skill to the appropriate use of questions, and indeed all forms of communication, is active listening. This involves knowing what your purpose is within the interaction, making a 100% commitment to achieve it, actively being aware of your tuning-in and tuning-out mechanisms, having the confidence in your ability to listen and handle whatever comes back, and, most important of all, believing in the client's right to be heard; in other words, hearing what they say afresh each time they come to see you.

A useful way of checking that you have heard what your client has said – and not what you think they have said – is to feed back the information that you have been given (an issue we covered in Ch. 5). You will find it extremely helpful in this process to use the client's own language, as this is a clear indicator to your client that she or he is being heard.

In repeating what you have heard, you will give your client time to think again about whether there is anything further that they wish to add. It also leaves them free of pressure in terms of having to come up with the 'right' answers or having to come up with explanations as to their behaviour. It is during this part of the process that you can use such phrases as:

'So, just how did you find it an enjoyable experience?'

'What was it do you think that left you feeling so upset?'

'How do you think you would like to improve the situation?

'What do you feel might help you to improve the situation?'

'What kind of resources do you think you would need to assist you?'

All open-ended questions are designed to help the client to think through and to make their own decisions. We feel that the aim of any therapy is that the client should leave the treatment room with more options and a greater feeling of well-being than when they entered it. To do this the client always needs to feel that they are in control of their life, and/or gaining more control over their life, and that they are being assisted by you and the treatment. All your questions, therefore, need to be on the basis of what and how, and not why.

Non-verbal communication

Let us now go on to the subject of body language – non-verbal communication. Many books have been written on the subject of body language and many categorical statements have been made regarding certain body postures denoting certain feelings or behaviour states.

The note of caution that we would draw here is to remind therapists that everybody is unique and that in the early stages of the therapist/client relationship you are learning to understand your client and learning about what some of their behaviours and mannerisms may denote. It is important to remember, however, that as your client changes and grows so their body language may also change and grow.

Active listening is communicated primarily through non-verbal means. It means not letting yourself drift off, however often you think you have heard the story before – the Americans call it 'staying tuned in'. It means watching your client for changes in body posture, facial and muscle tone, colour and expression. It means being attentive to voice tone, pauses, changes in pace of speech, hesitations, repetitions, metaphors etc. It means reflecting back what you have seen and checking out possible meanings.

Having emphasised this, we will now give you some pointers to aid you in understanding more about non-verbal communication. Do remember, however, that non-verbal communication is just one piece of information and does not stand alone, but needs to be taken in conjunction with the verbal communication that you are being given.

Starting from the top, the eyes. In neurolinguistic programming (NLP), eye movements are known as 'accessing cues'. Certain eye movements have been found to happen in particular ways when people are mentally searching for information (Fig. 7.1). Learning about these accessing cues gives you an understanding of your client's inner thought processes. Certain eye movements will reliably indicate that the client is gaining access to ideas or experiences in a *visual* way. Others will denote the accessing of information via *auditory* means, and others that the client is accessing the information through feelings and emotional responses, i.e. *kinesthetically*. (A client whose eye movements show a visual process will be helped to be put at ease if you demonstrate via your language that you have a capacity to 'see the world as they do', or that what they are saying 'really paints a picture' for you. But more of that under the section on 'language'.)

Where your client's eyes are directed when they are in conversation with you will help you to understand their own inner map of reality, and whether or not it is in conflict with the words that they are actually using. It will also aid you in pacing your client and matching their inner world through your use of language. (Should you wish to learn more about NLP, a useful introductory book is *Principles of NLP* by J O'Connor and I McDermott: Thorsens, 1996.)

Having possession of such information does not mean that you confront everything that your client is stating, but that you acknowledge where they are at this moment in time and give thought to the best way to work with them, now and in the future. Non-verbal information allows you to be more sensitive to the needs of your client; it is not permission to go crashing in.

Moving down the body, the next interesting piece of non-verbal communication is the use of the hands. You will note that when people are talking to you they often use their hands to emphasise or punctuate. You may also have heard the expression: 'Cut off my hands and I wouldn't be able to speak'. Most of us use our hands to illustrate what we are saying and you may find it particularly helpful to be able to read and understand this illustration. Watch in particular if a person touches a part of their body when they are in discussion with you.

A common illustration of this is when people are talking about things that are deeply painful to them or others – they will frequently touch their heart area. People who are expressing how uncomfortable they would feel trying to explain something to a superior, making a presentation, or giving a talk or speech will frequently touch their throat, collar or mouth.

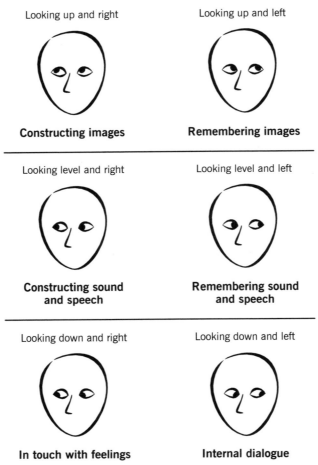

Looking up and right

Constructing images

Looking up and left

Remembering images

Looking level and right

Constructing sound
and speech

Looking level and left

Remembering sound
and speech

Looking down and right

In touch with feelings

Looking down and left

Internal dialogue

Figure 7.1 Clients' eye movements can give you access to their inner thought processes.

Your client may often exhibit signs of discomfort or unease by playing with their rings, watch, bracelet, neck jewellery or earrings. Discomfort or unease at disclosing information could result in looking away when they are talking to you, looking down towards the floor and not sitting still or looking relaxed.

A part of the body that is often overlooked in terms of non-verbal communication is the feet. On the surface, a client who is sitting comfortably in their chair with either their legs crossed or their feet on the ground could give the impression of being relaxed in their surroundings. In her book *The Bodymind Workbook* (Element Publishers), Debbie Shapiro states that if '...both feet [are] turned outwards, then there may be some confusion about where we are going; if our feet are turned inwards, then it can be saying that we are unclear in our direction'.

What it is important to remember in all of the above illustrations is that this is just one piece of one person's behaviour and before any inference can be drawn it needs to be viewed in the total context of the person, their environment and the other information that you are receiving. Does it all fit together; in other words, is it congruent?

What we do know is that our body language is by and large the most honest indicator of how we are feeling. Internalised tension will be demonstrated in body posture and movement. The secret of being able to perceive this information is to engage your client in an interesting conversation. What this does is to take their mind, i.e. their concentration, away from trying to control their body and from thinking about what they are saying to you. Once this happens, the body will adopt the posture that feels right for where it is at that particular moment. Once this has happened, you will be able to read – depending on your own brand of therapy – what the body is telling you.

Language

As discussed earlier, it is also important to listen to the type of language that is used. Is the person using metaphors that are visual, auditory or kinesthetic? Examples of each of these are:

◆ Visual

- 'I can't see it clearly.'

- 'It's all out of perspective.'

- 'Everybody looked through me.'

◆ Auditory

- 'That sounded strange to me.'

- 'That rings bells for me.'

- 'I don't think I heard him right.'

◆ Kinesthetic

- 'My heart sinks when...'

- 'It's a weight on my shoulders.'

- 'They froze me out.'

- 'It feels strange to me.'

You will aid your client by pacing their language, for example:

◆ Visual

  – 'I can see what you are saying.'

  – 'Can you picture a long-term solution?'

◆ Auditory

  – 'Can you tune into this idea?'

  – 'How does it sound to you?'

◆ Kinesthetic

  – 'How will you balance this with other demands?'

  – 'Did you get a feel for it?'

It is important that you convey understanding and non-judgmental acceptance of whatever your client wishes to tell you. You will need to demonstrate through your own body posture, verbal tone, head-nods, 'uh-huhs' etc. that you are listening and respecting what you are being told.

Here are some 'what-not-to' examples:

  'Don't you think that was a silly thing to do?'

  'That sounds rather unwise.'

  'I wonder why you did that?'

  'Oh my goodness!'

  'You didn't, did you?'

  'Why did you do that?'

accompanied by:

◆ avoiding eye contact

◆ locking eyes

◆ indifferent expression.

Making sense of information

Having gleaned all your information, you now need to make sense of it. Ask yourself:

◆ Is there a pattern appearing?

◆ Is there a body link as against an emotional link?

◆ Does the client want a change?

◆ Are there new factors emerging, and do they make sense yet?

◆ Is the client self-aware?

◆ Has the last treatment made any difference? In whose view?

◆ Is there a clear sense of where to go next?

When the pieces of verbal and non-verbal information that you have received are not in harmony, then you are faced with choices as to how you utilise the information. You will be guided in this by thinking about what it is you want to achieve on behalf of your client. How you present such information to your client is as vital to their health and well-being as collecting and collating such information. It is not an exercise in proving to your client how clever you are at retrieving information, but an offer to aid the client to develop more choices to deal with their particular issue.

Examples of good practice in this area could be:

'It is interesting that when you…talked about/mentioned/demonstrated/showed me, you…'

'Have you ever noticed that…?'

'What do you think that this might be about?'

'Do you think it is significant that…?'

'Do you think there is any relationship between…?'

'I wonder if…?'

'Do you think it is connected with…?'

'Do you think there is a connection between…?'

'Do you think that is because…?'

'Why do you feel that might be?' (Sometimes important to tune into the feelings as against the thoughts.)

'I had noticed that when we talk about X, Y seems to happen. What do you think this might be about?'

All of the above examples provide space for the client to think about issues and come to their own decisions as to where the links may be. Such questions do not put pressure on the client to perform or come up with the 'right' answers. It is important to remember that you are not a mind reader; you have a bodywork skill that your client wishes you to employ in order to assist them in dealing with whatever their problem or concern may be. You are the expert in your field, and the client is the expert in his or her own field. Your client will have approached you and sought information as to whether or not your particular therapy, and its particular application, was what they required. You in turn will be involved in assisting your client to provide as much information as possible to aid you in carrying out your task. The secret of this process is to encourage your client to do the talking, at both a verbal and a non-verbal level. Your role in this process is to encourage, clarify where necessary, and ask the kind of questions that allow your client not only to think about issues but also to view them from a different perspective.

A useful model for you to follow is that of Gerard Egan. This is a three stage model, and one that we have found provides a simple and clear framework. Gerard Egan – along with others – believed that clients and their therapists should focus on goals. In the three stage model:

> In stage one the helper's goal is responding, whereas the client's goal is self-exploration. In stage two the helper's goal is integrative understanding, whereas the client's goal is dynamic understanding. In stage three, the helper's goal is facilitating action, whereas the client's goal is acting.

Put simply, the role of the therapist in the first stage is to encourage the client to tell their story with minimal interruption: 'Tell me about...'. In stage two, the therapist is assisting the client to 'make sense' of issues and to examine them from different perspectives: 'What does that say to you now?' In stage three, the therapist is facilitating the client in action: 'What would you need for that to happen?'

You can use this model to guide your 'first 10 minutes' of each session, and also use it as a framework to plot the total treatment process.

Having started to make sense of the information, it is important that you do not allow this 10 minute session to turn into one of counselling. It is therefore vital that you always hold in the forefront of your mind the purpose of the session, i.e. how current issues are affecting the client's physical system and how these can be helped through the session's treatment. You will need to be disciplined about managing this period of time, what it is meant to achieve and what it is not meant to achieve, i.e. a counselling process.

Throughout this period (and indeed for the whole treatment), it is important that the client feels in control of what is happening to them. Therefore, the more understanding and knowledge that they have about the treatment, and the need for the kind of questions that you will be asking, the more relaxed and forthcoming they are likely to be. None of us likes to expose too much of ourselves without being clear about what the information is going to be used for!

Preparing the client for the primary treatment

To round off this part of the treatment, you will find it useful to summarise what your client has told you and to reinforce how the treatment can assist:

'So, you're saying that … and that suggests that today we need to…'

'What I have heard you telling me is … and what you're telling me you need is…'

'So if this … is still a problem, I think today we should…'

Your client will then be able to move into the next part of the treatment process confident in the knowledge that what is important to them has been heard by their therapist and will be reflected in the treatment.

> In this chapter, we have stressed the importance of the therapist becoming a skilled communicator, fully understanding and utilising their own verbal and non-verbal skills and being aware of the verbal and non-verbal information emanating from the client. Good communication is a skill that can be learned, and good communicators keep on acquiring new skills. The secret is to keep on learning and to keep on practising! As Bert Decker reminds us in his book *How to communicate effectively* (Kogan Page), 'communicating well is a lifetime process'.

8 Managing the unexpected

When something happens that falls outside what we expect, we often feel threatened or alarmed. All human beings work much of the time predicting on the basis of past experience – after all, this saves us from endless wondering about small things. One of the most alarming moments in Tolkien's *The Lord of the Rings*, just before the last battle with the Dark Lord, was when the sun *didn't* rise in the morning. All skill learning relies on a substantial amount of learned expectation: if I do this, that will result; this approach, or this substance, is effective for that condition. Even where we build in qualifications like 'normally' and 'usually', we often have a back-up expectation as well – if this doesn't work, that may be effective; if the client doesn't respond like this, they may respond like that.

But what if something occurs that is outside what we could have foreseen? This is a potentially alarming, even threatening, experience for both therapist and client. This chapter offers a model which can help to distinguish between different kinds of unexpected behaviour, so that the therapist is in a better position to respond helpfully, even where the reasons for the behaviour are puzzling or unknown.

> You are in the middle of a massage, and so far the client has seemed very comfortable and relaxed. Suddenly they shudder and burst into tears. Or perhaps you are taking notes in a first consultation: the client is attentive and cooperative, answering your questions quite readily. You may even be looking down to make notes while asking the next routine question. There is a pause: you look up and find the client flushed, with watering eyes and trembling lip. What is going on? What do you do?

You may even be wondering what you have done to provoke such a reaction. Most of the time, this will not be the case. But even if you feel the reaction was provoked by a lack of skill on your part, the immediate need is to manage the situation as it is. If you really feel you need to apologise, do it, but don't grovel. Even the most experienced professionals make mistakes at times. Above all, focus on what needs to happen now to retrieve the situation, not on what an idiot you feel. Calmly taking control of the situation and remedying it goes a long way to restoring the client's confidence. They may see you as an expert, but most people are generous enough – and realistic enough – to know that even experts don't get it right all the time.

The reactions we have described are marked physical events which seem unrelated in content and degree to what is 'actually' going on. Yet, as a wise colleague once said: 'There is no reaction, however bizarre, that doesn't have some meaning to the person themselves.' Sometimes the client will know and volunteer the meaning there and then: 'I'm sorry, that piece of music was my mother's favourite', or 'It's not your fault, but asking about brothers and sisters hit a raw nerve; you see we had a major family row a few weeks ago...'. More puzzling are reactions which even the client can't understand: 'I don't know what that was about: I just suddenly felt cold all over', or 'Goodness me, I can't think what's upset me like this.'

Sometimes a mismatch between what is ongoing and the client's behaviour may be less immediately obvious. You ask a question and the client begins to answer. After a few moments you realise they have drifted off the subject. You bring them back again, and again they deflect. Or they may tell you about something you think they would find distressing, yet they are smiling. You are doing some bodywork and suddenly there is a burst of giggles.

It may be useful here to show a model developed many years ago and used a lot in social work and psychotherapy training. It's known as the Johari Window (named, some say, after two men, Joe and Harry, who invented it!) (see Fig. 8.1).

Unexpected client behaviour may fall into any of these categories:

1. Neither the client nor the therapist knows what caused the behaviour.

2. The client knows the cause but the therapist doesn't

3. The client isn't aware of the cause but the therapist is (or may have a shrewd idea).

4. Both client and therapist are aware of the cause.

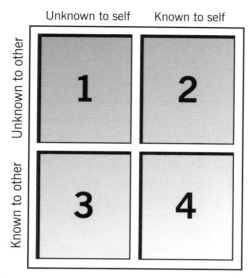

Figure 8.1 The Johari Window.

1. Where neither party knows the cause

Both are likely to be startled and both may be alarmed. In this case, the therapist needs to be accepting. You are in charge of the client and their welfare in your treatment room, and it is your responsibility to help them with what happens there.

Don't ignore what happened. Pause in what you are doing unless it's absolutely impossible (in that case, stop as soon as you can). Ask them what would be most helpful right now. Depending on the client and your relationship with them, you could then stay silent but close, ask if they want a blanket or towel (sudden emotional responses often make people feel chilled), or a hand or a shoulder to cry on. *Don't do any of these things without asking and without consent:* you don't know what is going on for the client and it is important to give them time and space. Their reaction is an important response and may be the source of important learning or change.

Don't leap to reassure the client. You don't know what is going on, so resist the temptation to say, 'It's all right'. It probably doesn't feel like that to the client, so saying it creates an incongruity and distance between you. Your manner can be reassuring, but it's too early to know whether your words should.

Where a reaction like this is profound or extensive, it is called an *abreaction*. One of our tutors, advising student therapists on dealing with abreactions, used to say that the best response was to 'sit back and shut up'. The reaction belongs to the client: all they need initially from you is permission and support.

Later – maybe in minutes – they may be ready to talk about it. When their words or action tell you that they are 'back again' and reorientated, you may tell them that there must be a good reason for their reaction and that at some point its meaning is likely to become clear to them. Let them know that they needn't apologise – this is not an uncommon happening. If they seem to want to discuss it, or to speculate about causes, follow their lead. Ask them if they want to abandon the rest of the physical treatment you had planned, or if they would like a drink or just to be quiet for a few minutes.

Sometimes these kinds of abreactions may involve emotion: other times, they may involve a marked physical response but little or no feeling. These are often very puzzling to both client and therapist. In our experience, such marked reactions with an absence of emotion may indicate that the client has unconsciously connected with a major, often childhood, trauma at a physical level, but that they are unconsciously protecting themselves against emotional recall. (The most obvious, but not the only, example of this is where the client has been sexually abused in childhood.) *Do not suggest to the client that this may be the case.* You could ask them if they feel as though their reaction belongs to the present, or more as if it connects with something in the past. It can be helpful to remember that when we are upset we often feel much younger than our chronological age. Sometimes it can be helpful to ask, when something like this happens, 'How old do you feel at the moment?' Remind them that our bodies hold a store of experience as well as our brains (why practise your golf swing if they don't!) and that something may have connected on that level.

Being upset makes us feel out of control, because we have not been able to disguise our feelings. It can be upsetting to become aware of a feeling we had not previously recognised in ourselves, but when that response happens in front of someone else it usually feels even worse.

Even if the reaction does not connect with the past in any way, we are likely to lose contact for a while with the competent adult part of ourselves. Allowing a client time to recover from such an experience also allows them to reconnect with this coping part and to shift from raw feeling towards a more analytic/left brain state which can begin to take charge again.

If the client does seem emotionally upset, ask if they know someone they could talk to about how they feel. Suggest the name of a counsellor if their response indicates they don't already know someone they can trust, or would feel embarrassed about talking to someone they already know.

2. Known to client: not known to therapist

This one is more straightforward, since the client is aware of what provoked the response. The initial response of pausing, allowing and offering can be the same. The client may volunteer information (as in our examples). Or you can say: 'Would you like to talk about that?' If the response is negative, you can ask, as before, if they have someone they trust or if they would like you to suggest someone. Again, you may need to abandon or curtail your plans for the rest of the session, doing only what is essential so that you and the client have time to pick up the pieces. The client needs to go out of your treatment room feeling able to face the world again. If they are very shaken, it may help to offer them a cup of tea, coffee or water and some time in your waiting/sitting room. If you have Rescue Remedy, this may be the time to offer it.

If you have another client following on immediately, suggest the first client lets themselves out when they feel ready. Alternatively, call them a cab or let them phone a friend or family member to collect them if they don't feel able to face driving or public transport.

3. Known to therapist: unknown to client

In your training, you will have learnt that bodywork can sometimes provoke certain reactions and that clients may not expect them. These fall into two groups:

◆ *Reactions the client needs to be told about in advance.* If you know that the client is likely to react in a certain way as a result of your treatment, warn them. Even gentle hands-on work can sometimes leave the client feeling exhausted or very sore. If this is probable, tell them so that they can plan their next few hours or days around it. If a reaction might happen, but might not, or if there are several possible reactions, tell them the possibilities. Clients may expect physical reactions to physical treatment, but are unlikely to expect increased feelings of emotional fragility, or irritability, so it can be helpful to say: 'Some people feel edgy after this kind of work, so if you should be one of them just tell your family it isn't your fault and ask them to make allowances for a day or two.'

◆ *Reactions that may be provoked by expectation.* The human animal is distinguished by the ability to anticipate. This is an essential and valuable skill, but we want to avoid building in happenings that don't have to happen. Sometimes, and with some clients in particular, you may need to hold back from telling them that they might feel or react in a certain way because of the risk that they will make it happen. Jerome K. Jerome's *Three Men in a Boat* begins with an account of how the hero looked up some of his symptoms in a medical dictionary, went on reading and became convinced that he had every ailment in the book apart from housemaid's knee. Self-dramatising clients are particularly prone to this kind of thing.

Assessing the probability of a self-induced reaction, and weighing it up against the advisability of preparing the client for something which, if it did happen, could be disconcerting, unpleasant or undermining of confidence in the therapy or therapist is not always easy. It may be easier to tell the client that it is very unlikely that they will experience an adverse reaction to the treatment, but that they can phone you if they do. Some clients will also understand you if you explain that you do not want them to be looking unnecessarily for further symptoms! Bear in mind the rather difficult principle that if we once mention something we raise the possibility of it in the client's mind. How many patients didn't think of discomfort until the nurse or doctor said: 'This shouldn't hurt.' What shouldn't it do? *HURT*.

In other words, only warn against what is probable, or what, if it were to occur, would be alarming.

4. Known to client and known to therapist

Reactions in this category, however marked, tend to be the least alarming. One or other of you, after the initial surprise, is likely to say something like: 'Well, I can see why that happened, can't you?' Taking a good case history at the outset, and regular notes as the case progresses, will have given you lots of information about the client. When they react in a marked manner, whether physically or emotionally, cast your mind back to the moment when things changed. What was being done or discussed? Something was a trigger, something made a connection, set off a response. Rewind your tape of the last few minutes; consult your mental file on this client; look for key words, actions. Scan for changes of posture, changes of colour in your replay. Being attentive, you are likely to have noticed the beginnings of changes, even though the speed of transition to a major reaction may have caught you unawares.

Finding the key word or action may give you a clue to the meaning even before you or the client mentions it. It may be that in scanning you remember a less extreme but similar reaction some time in the past – in other words, you become aware that there is a pattern here which you had not registered before. This can be useful information. You may want to discuss it with the client or file it away for future reference.

Overall, the best advice we can give was given to us by one of our tutors in training: *think on your feet*. You have many skills relevant to this situation. You have your professional training, you have your life skills, you have human empathy and concern. You have a valuable toolbag of experience and knowledge. Something in there will be relevant or can be adapted.

Take a deep breath. Focus on the client's situation. Remind yourself that being respectfully attentive gives you the best chance of finding out what they need right now, and that analysis, learning and future planning can all come later. Say what you see – 'That seems rather distressing for you'; 'You look uncomfortable'; 'You're shivering' – and ask: 'Is there anything you would like me to do?' Reflecting what you see affirms the reality of the client's experience: asking what they would like you to do puts them back in control of the situation (even if their reply is: 'What do you think is best?' – that's a choice to defer to your expertise). The implicit message for the client is that even the unexpected can be managed. That's an important therapeutic learning in itself.

We have looked in this chapter at different kinds of unexpected situations which may occur in therapy, and at some ways to make our responses appropriately and supportively. We have a range of instinctive, as well as trained, ways of reacting to what is unpredicted, and sometimes need to hold back on the impulse to reassure and comfort while continuing to 'hold' the client with a professional support. We believe that the difference between amateurism and professionalism in these situations is rather like that between sympathy and empathy. The amateur may be *sympathetic* – in other words they identify or 'feel with' the person suffering. The professional is *empathic*, i.e. makes an imaginative effort to understand what may be going on for the client without being sucked into the feeling themselves. Only when we can show understanding without sharing the client's pain, helplessness or alarm can we be truly helpful to them. Once we join them, we cease to be of value to them – most of all, in situations which surprise us both.

9 Reorientating the client and ending the session

Ending the session and enabling the client to leave with a sense of calmness and completeness are fundamental to effective treatment.

This chapter will cover the five stage process of reorientating and ending a treatment session:

◆ Mind-set – encouraging and supporting change

◆ Expectations and instructions

◆ Payment

◆ Future treatments

◆ Separating and saying goodbye.

Mind-set

The hands-on component of the treatment is now complete and the client is about to enter the next phase of treatment: the realisation that change – sometimes at many levels – has taken place.

Because all forms of bodywork involve the client in some form of dislocation from their normal state of being, to a new or altered state, there may need to be assistance to orientate to this new state, and to reorientate actions, behaviours and attitudes outside the treatment room.

With such therapies as osteopathy, acupuncture or sports injury massage, a physical state has been changed and the client may well need assistance to adjust to the new/altered state: this may involve emotional as well as physical adjustment. With therapies such as aromatherapy and reflexology, an emotional and/or physical state is altered, and again there will be a period of orientating to the new state.

So what is the role of the therapist in this process? How do they communicate information about this process of adjustment that will put the client into a fit state to take control of their life emotionally and physically, but not leave them anxious and nervous about how they will manage? The secret lies in *when* and *how* the information is given.

The action of going to see a bodywork therapist is a desire for some form of change to take place, it is also an action of trust. In effect the client hands over control of all or part of their body, in order that the therapist can use their skills and knowledge to contribute to a change. The process of handing back the control starts when the client is told, in some form or another: 'I will now leave you to get dressed.' It is at this stage, often with the client totally relaxed, the trust still with the therapist and *before they have started dressing*, that the therapist can start the reorientating process by skilful use of presuppositions. For example:

'You may still find yourself holding your arm stiffly. This is only natural, and **you will forget** *all about it within a day or two.'*

'You may feel a little light-headed as you get up. This is nothing to worry about **and will pass** *in a few minutes.'*

'I would like you *to take 5 minutes now to* **further relax** *and* **plan how you will take this state of relaxation** *with you into your everyday busy schedule.'*

'...realising that it may take **a few days for you to feel even better than you do now.'***

'Initially as you dress you may still find it a little painful, **but this will disappear** *in a couple of days.'*

 Jot down a few phrases that you could use that would be appropriate in your therapy.

Expectations and instructions

Whilst the client is dressing, you can update your records and check your notes to see if there is any specific guidance or instruction needed, e.g. home study, therapeutic exercise etc. Do be aware that your client may well take longer to dress than they did to undress, and allow for this.

Once the client is dressed, it will be important to reaffirm and/or summarise the treatment and some of the probable effects that they might experience in the days following treatment:

'It may be that over the next few days you will ... but this will pass.'

'Some people experience a slight headache, but it does not normally last more than a few hours.'

It will also be important for you to check with your client how they are feeling, and make sure that they are comfortable with this. If this is not the case then provide them with; (1) an awareness of what has happened to cause the feeling; (2) how long it is likely to last; (3) reassurance that all is well. For example:

'The reason you may be feeling like this is because.... This is a perfectly normal reaction after such a treatment and nothing for you to worry about. In a few ... it will have passed.'

It is at this stage of the treatment that you need to be clear with your client about the taking or otherwise of medication, strenuous exercise, helpful exercises, suggested relaxation techniques etc. – in other words, what are necessary, acceptable and unacceptable behaviours, and what might happen concerning the effects of the treatment if they disregard your advice (once again handing the control back to the client). It is helpful for you to support this with written material and instructions. (It also means that there is no danger of the client forgetting what they have been told once they leave your treatment rooms.)

Payment and future treatments

In most cases, these two actions take place almost simultaneously. Once you and your client have finished discussing current treatment, the next step is payment and future appointments. If the treatment is not yet completed then you will need to be specific: 'I need to see you in ... days/weeks.' If it is being left to the client's discretion then either of 'When would you like to come again?' or 'Would you like to come again?' leaves the client free to make the decision. They may of course seek your advice, being unsure what the norm is, in which case use your knowledge of the client and their case history to inform your answer.

If during this process the client has not given you your fee, then a simple 'That will be £x.xx for today's session please' will be a natural link to your previous conversation.

Separating and saying goodbye

Having assured yourself that your client is now ready to leave and assuming you are satisfied that this is the case, it may be that you need to mark this juncture by rising from your chair. (Some clients become so immersed in their treatment that they lose all track of time.) Such a move signals firmly yet politely that the session has ended. As you rise to your feet and escort them to the door, it will be useful to reaffirm the next appointment: 'Goodbye Ms Q, have a good week, and I will look forward to seeing you on the ... at ....'

If this is your last appointment with your client, then recapping on their situation when they first came to you, and their progress up to this point, marks the process you have been through and the changes that have taken place. It is also a fitting way to end the treatment – on a positive note.

If a client is ending treatment at a stage when you feel more work would be beneficial, still go through the above process, as it allows them to leave feeling positive and able to return for treatment at some further stage. Do tell them that you wish them well, that you have enjoyed working with them and that you are always happy to see former clients who might want new or additional treatment.

Bringing the treatment to an effective close involves not compromising the effectiveness of your work by rushing your client. Although the ending of the session is usually brief, it too conveys implicit messages to the client. It will be important to take time and care to ensure that the messages are those of calm completion, forward-looking confidence, continued respect for self and, if appropriate, availability of further treatment in the future.

> As we stated at the beginning of the chapter: 'Ending the session and enabling the client to leave with a sense of calmness is fundamental to effective treatment.' It is also fundamental to the process continuing outside the treatment room. Effective therapy is a process, not an event, and how a client receives messages concerning their future well-being will have an impact on the effectiveness of that process. Each part of the treatment process is vital to the care and well-being of the client, and none more so than the final stage of reorientating and bringing the treatment session to an accomplished conclusion.

3

Managing your practice: effective administration and dealing with common client issues

Contents

10 Where to practise

You need a place in which to practise. Essentially, there are three possibilities (or a combination of them):

◆ your home

◆ a clinic

◆ the client's home.

In this chapter, we are going to work through some of the features of each, looking at what may be advantages and disadvantages. This is another question of matching, because you need to be at ease and to find your workplace congenial and conducive to offering your best. What suits one therapist may not suit another. What bothers one therapist may not bother another at all. But envisioning yourself in various kinds of possible settings, and doing some preparatory homework before making a commitment, will pay off.

Finding the right environment

Some issues are practical, some are more to do with how we feel. But practicalities also convey messages, both to you and to your client, as we have emphasised throughout. Our surroundings have a powerful effect on us – our comfort, our well-being, our ability to concentrate. Some buildings are even 'toxic' (a term now in frequent use). Remember that whereas the client will only be in your workplace for an hour or two, you might be there all day, 5 days a week (and perhaps some evenings too). Your setting really matters!

The context of therapeutic work also conveys messages to the client and may affect their choice of therapist. Some people undoubtedly prefer visiting a therapist in the therapist's home, while some feel safer or think that treatment is more 'professional' in a clinic. Others feel more comfortable (or can spare the time more easily) if you visit them. There are plenty of clients to go round, and you will find that whichever option you choose will draw people who are as comfortable there as you are.

So in evaluating these possibilities, we have both the therapist and the client in mind, and are looking at factors which range from the very practical or obvious to the implicit, and from short-term to long-term in their effects.

Working from home

Take a look at your home. Imagine you are a potential client. If you have already thought of working at home, you are likely to have thought about whether you have a suitable spare room or whether you could convert a dining room or conservatory. So you will already have begun the process of imagining a new reality – constructing a future.

Walk around your home, starting with the front door. Be a client. Where will you have to go? What will you pass, or pass through, in order to get there? In looking through a client's eyes, you are likely to see some things you have taken for granted or learned to ignore. What about the pile of shoes behind the front door, and the shopping bag hanging on the sitting room door handle? What will they make of the playgroup collage or your choice of posters? Whatever the objects, be sure they will make something of what they see – and will totally overlook some other things which to you look equally obvious (or more obvious). We go into these things in more detail in the next chapter.

In assessing the practicalities for the client of working at home, it is important to plot their route, from arrival to departure, and to see how easy and comfortable it could be made or what problems it might present. They will need:

◆ access to a lavatory

◆ somewhere to wait

   – if early

   – while waiting to be collected

   – if you overrun with an earlier client.

If you are going to treat people whose mobility is limited by reason of infirmity, disability or age, is your treatment room accessible to them? If it is upstairs (converted spare bedroom – a favourite choice), do you have an alternative, downstairs room you could work by arrangement, or will you have to check with potential clients that they can manage stairs?

Many clients come by car. Is there easy parking?

How easy would it be for you to make your house into your workplace ? You will need to think about:

◆ designating and equipping a room

◆ readying it at the beginning of a working day

◆ ensuring privacy

◆ preventing interruptions

◆ keeping everyday life (which may include hobbies, partners, children and pets) at an appropriate distance.

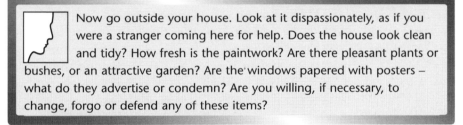

Now go outside your house. Look at it dispassionately, as if you were a stranger coming here for help. Does the house look clean and tidy? How fresh is the paintwork? Are there pleasant plants or bushes, or an attractive garden? Are the windows papered with posters – what do they advertise or condemn? Are you willing, if necessary, to change, forgo or defend any of these items?

Some clients will be delighted by the way you vote; others will not notice. Yet others may feel you are the wrong sort of person to help them because of your political views. Our point is not that you have to be all things to all people; only that clients will – and must – make something of the information which confronts them, and it is up to us to decide whether any of that potential information gets in the way of our therapy. If so, would it hurt to modify it?

The advantages of working from home

The atmosphere is more personal

Many clients feel much more comfortable in someone's home. If lacking confidence (which is very common), they may find it easier to confide or relax. They may like your personal style even if it is different from their own. We have known clients to enjoy our friendly clutter of ornaments and pictures even though they said they personally had to have bare, spare, tidy surfaces in their own homes. In non-medical therapies, clients often feel more at ease knowing something about their therapist as a person – even if that is only what can be gleaned from surroundings rather than from personal information. Most of us have a degree of curiosity about other people's homes, and clients can sometimes find interests or tastes in common which helps them feel more at ease.

The surroundings are more informal

When people are ill or distressed, they can sometimes feel less fragile in a more personal atmosphere. What they see around them may also give opportunities for small talk which can ease the stress of becoming a client or meeting a new person.

Your time can be more flexible

If you stay in the house to work, you have more non-work time available because you don't have to travel. You can also use the time in between appointments for other things, and if, sadly, a client cancels at the last moment, or fails to turn up (though we intend to help you ensure that these are only very infrequent and unavoidable occurrences), then you are not stuck waiting somewhere with nothing else to do except feel frustrated and angry, or disappointed. You can fill in with domestic tasks, do other work related to your therapy, or sit with your feet up. This flexibility can be particularly useful when you first start in practice, before your diary gets really busy.

Home is less intimidating

Clients are often afraid of being vulnerable. It can be difficult to discuss personal or physical difficulties, particularly if this is the first time one has asked for help. Hospitals and doctors' surgeries may have left the client feeling intimidated by professionals. No one seems too official in their own home with their own things around them. This is a powerful advantage. We have often found that our pets help clients relax, and have enjoyed visiting other therapists, when we have been clients ourselves, who also have pets. With talking therapies, pets may helpfully stay in the treatment room if the client agrees. With body therapies they are probably best kept to waiting areas, but they can still put people at ease.

You can do your own telephone contact and sifting of potential clients

As Chapter 3 shows, there are lots of advantages to making your own bookings. At home, you can do this quite flexibly, provided you ensure that you are not at the mercy of answering each and every phonecall there and then.

If you have young children it is easier to work at home

Working for yourself from home is the ultimate in flexibility. If you have young children, you can arrange your working hours around the school run times. If you want to attend the school play, help with swimming or a school trip, you can take time out from work and rearrange your diary for that week. Since many therapists train as a second career, they often do have young families, and working at home makes the transition easier.

You can make use of the time when clients don't turn up

Being at home also eases the sense of anxiety which comes from having relatively few clients at the outset of practice, or at 'thin' times of year like January and August. It is easier not to feel threatened by the lack of clients when you are working at home rather than when renting premises and having to pay for them anyway at these times. It takes time to become confident that there is enough work out there and that it will come to you; and when we are anxious all the pressures of the job get to us more. If you are in a clinic and a client fails to turn up, you may have to find things to do until the time of the next appointment, while around you the colleagues who share the building seem to be busy with their clients. This can be very dispiriting. It is easier to distract yourself at home by finding something else to do – and sometimes one is genuinely glad to have an extra hour or two for some project or task.

If you work at home, it may make sense to actively decide to take your own holidays when work is thinnest. If many of your clients are women with their own young children, you could elect to have a holiday at half-terms, and in part of the Easter holiday, as well as taking the more usual breaks at Christmas and in the summer. (You will need to take account of this in your financial planning, so as to save some income for your lean times.)

Disadvantages of working from home

It can be distracting

You will need to get into work mode in working hours at home. This means either ensuring that home needs and tasks are done before you begin work or finding a way to put the thought of them aside even if something unexpectedly reminds you. Having a work room helps, of course, because everything there is focused on your work and your clients' needs. Have a jotter handy in case any non-work need or task occurs to you, so that at some point you can scribble down a key word and free your professional attention from things which don't belong.

What do you do if someone knocks at the door? If at all possible, ignore them – after all, you wouldn't be able to answer if you were out. If you have regular working hours, let your immediate neighbours know (if you are friendly with them) so that they don't interrupt you. If you have older children who can be left on their own when you are working, make sure they know what you want them to do about callers – should they ignore the knock, or are they old enough and sensible enough to open the door and deal with the caller?

If the phone rings, of course the answerphone will deal with it, and you may like to tell your client before you start work that it is on and that you do not intend answering the door unless there is some unusual and unanticipated reason.

You need to dedicate a room to your therapy

It is not feasible to do regular therapy in a room which has another use. It takes too much time to reorganise from one use to another and there are too many possibilities of forgetting something. It doesn't impress the client if you have to search for an oil you want for their treatment, which somehow got left out of the box when you last put it away, or if you have to find the paper roll for the couch – now where did that go? The message, again, is not fully professional. You will probably be able to remember other examples from the time when you were training and practising with colleagues, family or friends in less than ideal settings.

So you will have to set aside a room just for your work – goodbye to the spare bedroom, the sewing room or the office, or even the junk room. This might be difficult if you are pressed for space. Long-term, you could think about converting a loft for that spare room, building on a conservatory or even buying another house – once you know your practice is succeeding. Perhaps your garden is big enough for a fair-sized summerhouse?

If you absolutely must use your treatment room for a spare room, don't leave a bed in it, as this carries confusing or unwanted messages. Get a sofabed or a futon with a base which can be used as a seat for the consultation part of your therapy, or keep a mattress in another room to bring in when needed for a guest.

You need an answerphone

We have enthused about the uses of answerphones before, so hopefully it will already seem like a good idea. However, it is an expense at the outset, and sometimes family and friends feel you are distancing them. We have received messages that said: 'Go on, answer! I know you're there!' You don't have to leave the answerphone on all the time, of course, although we actually feel this works better (see Ch. 3) and people do become accustomed to it.

What if your partner or child needed to get hold of you in an emergency? The easiest way to manage this is to agree some kind of family code, only to be used in such cases, e.g. getting the caller to put the phone down after it has rung less than the number of times needed for your machine to cut in, then ringing again at once. Whatever system you devise, *only tell this code to people who must have a means of reaching you urgently.*

You need somewhere for clients to wait

However punctual they are, some clients will arrive early or before the previous client has left. Buses or trains may be widely spaced, the weather may be too bad for even the most considerate of clients to walk around the block another time. If your sitting room isn't suitable, or is unavailable, could you put a chair in the hall? Remember, your client is likely to appreciate a magazine to look at.

The waiting area needs to be tidy and neutral. It is probably not appropriate to ask clients to wait in a sitting room where your teenage children and their friends are having coffee and chatting, or to sit in the background while small children have tea and watch television, though some clients won't mind. You need to plan an arrangement that will suit most of your clientele most of the time.

The house has to be tidy

All 'public' areas of your house have to be tidy when clients come. This means allowing enough time after people who live with you have got off to work or school in the morning to clear the debris – or to make sure that they do it – before the first client arrives. It could mean checking last thing at night that the sitting room is tidy for the following day. It might mean more frequent dusting and vacuuming of public areas, rather than allowing a friendly tolerance of general pleasant disorder to develop between bouts of tidying. (It is pleasant, by contrast, to go into a clean, tidy, nice-smelling clinic where all this readying has been done by someone else – but then that is one of the things that you are having to pay for!)

Tidiness is not just visual. How will clients respond to the smell of curry, or garlic, from last night, or being prepared for tonight's supper? You may need to rearrange your menus accordingly. How might they feel about the smell of chip fat or cigarettes when they come in? Some won't mind, some will actively like the smells, while others might not want to come again. Clearly, it is easier to keep your treatment room free of unwanted or obtrusive smells than the kitchen or living room, but clients will have to go through some public areas first, and some smells may linger there.

Animals and children

Both are sources of varied reactions. Pets may help people relax. Children may bring out the best in the client. The general rule, however, needs to be that clients do not have to deal with either. Their primary purpose in being in your house is to receive your help via your therapy and your personal resourcefulness. You can ask in advance if you have any reason to think the client may be allergic, e.g. 'Are dogs a problem for you?' If the allergy is very severe, you may have to suggest that the client sees another therapist – or visit them in their home if you are prepared to do that. Or perhaps they will be able to cope if the dog is not in the waiting area when they come.

It goes without saying that, if you have small children, you need to make arrangements for them that leave you entirely free of responsibility for them while your clients are with you. Children of any age may need warning that they will have to be quieter than usual while you are working – no shouting, no loud stereo, no TV. This may require some bargaining if you work during evenings, after school hours or at weekends. It can also be harder to 'switch off' when small children are ill, even if you have someone with them.

Boundary-keeping may be more difficult

Pets and children bring up the issue of boundaries, which is another key area of concern for therapists in many ways and which we explore more fully in later chapters. Boundaries are often easier to keep when we actually go out to work, because the change of place keys us into our 'work-selves' and allows us more easily to leave our private selves at home. Being at home is a natural key into our private identities, so we have to make more deliberate effort. Having special work clothing (see Ch. 11) can help us change mode, and working in a special room reinforces it. We discuss elsewhere the need to protect our professional selves from being activated or exploited when we are off duty (see Ch. 12). It can be harder to remember which role we are in when we are new in practice, because our defences aren't so built up and our patterns not yet well established and automatic.

It's harder to leave work behind

This is another aspect of the boundary issue. Various tricks or mechanisms may help.

◆ If you have work clothes, change out of them as soon as you finish work.

◆ Shut your workroom door when you finish.

◆ Write up your client notes the same day, so you don't have information or concerns to carry over into private time until you have another time to write it down.

◆ Invent little rituals to make a break between work and non-work. Have a cup of coffee or another favourite drink. Have a shower or bath. Meditate or use another relaxation technique for a short while. Go for a walk or a jog.

If you have family responsibilities, or a partner coming home, you may be tempted to plunge straight into your other life when work finishes. Talk through with those around you the need for you to have a little buffer time to readjust – after all, people who went out to work have journeys home during which to change focus, and children have the trip home from school. Your need for a neutral time is as great as theirs, but unlike them you have no in-built activity or time to provide it. Experiment and find out what works.

There is extra wear and tear on furnishings and carpets

Having clients coming regularly into your home makes extra demands on your carpets and soft furnishings. (They also use up lavatory paper, soap and tissues.) Talk with your accountant about offsetting some of the necessary replacements or repairs against tax. This is a legitimate expense, but will have to be documented. You will also need advice on the best way to do this and on the implications for capital gains tax if you later sell a house/flat which has partially been used for business.

You may need to apply for a change of use

If you work from home, you may need to obtain permission from your local council for change of use, as the building is no longer solely being used as a domestic dwelling. This can sometimes be difficult. Some therapists risk not making the application: if your clients come sufficiently irregularly and so look like normal visitors, this may well save you trouble, since many body therapies are unlikely to cause disturbance to neighbours. Talk through the pros and cons with your accountant and with any other local therapists you know well who also practise from home.

Expenses and tax

If you rent a room to work from, the rent can be set down as a claimable expense of your business. If you work at home, it is more difficult to demonstrate which expenses are due to your business and which overlap with ordinary domestic needs. Seek advice, but work out how the house would be used and maintained if you were not working at home. How much gas/electricity did you use before? What is your consumption (or estimated consumption) now? Do you have to employ a cleaner now that you have strangers in your home? How many rooms in your house will clients need access to (include kitchen if they make drinks, lavatories/bathrooms, sitting room for waiting etc.). You can then work out a proportion of the household costs that relates to the proportion of the house used by clients. If you move house, you may have to pay back some of these offset costs, as the discounted tax would effectively have enabled you to make a personal profit. Talk with your accountant at the outset, so that from the beginning of your practice you do what is needed.

Additional capital outlay

If your room does not already have one, you may have to install a wash basin, and perhaps additional or different lighting. Curtains or blinds and heating may all need to be adjusted to cater for the needs of partially clothed clients. Having additional or separately controlled heating in your work room will help keep clients warm without roasting the others who live with you.

Working in a clinic

Reading through all the possible disadvantages of working at home may have set you up to feel that almost anywhere else is better! That choice may already have been made for you by external factors. You may not have a room that can be converted for your therapy. You may be living in rented property with a lease that makes it difficult or impossible to practise a business from home.

The obvious alternative is to rent a room somewhere, usually with another practitioner or group of practitioners in some kind of clinic setting. Let's consider the factors involved in this option.

Advantages

You get purpose-built or purpose-adapted premises

A clinic has usually been chosen for its setting, both in terms of accessibility for clients and in terms of the spaces it offers within. There is no trekking out into distant suburbs (if that is where you live) but usually somewhere central to the town or its main suburban areas, with relatively easy public transport access, perhaps even good parking on the street or even in a designated car park.

Inside, there will be a waiting area, toilets, a receptionist, a greater range of magazines than you would probably afford at home, perhaps also a box of toys for children to play with while they wait. There will be rooms set up with necessary basic equipment – sinks, lights, desks, filing cabinets. If you use a couch, the room may already come equipped with one. Carpets will have been chosen with a view to hard wear and possible spillages. The premises will probably be someone else's responsibility. Ideally, you will just have to walk in and work.

You get moral support from colleagues

For many, this is one of the major advantages. Working alone one-to-one can feel very lonely and unsupported for some therapists (others, however, love it). You will recently have been in a very supportive atmosphere where teachers and, above all, fellow students have been there for you in an emotional and practical sense. You could discuss queries and problems arising from your work and your practice clients; you could check out doubts about technique. You had someone to talk to about personal ups and downs. Relatively suddenly, you have become the person expected to provide support and guidance, knowledge and skill. You are *It*. In a clinic, there can be a real sense of comradely support, ranging from the unspoken sense of shared professionalism through to the ability to ask for information. There may be another practitioner of your therapy working there, if the clinic is relatively large, perhaps not on the same day as you, but at least available on the phone. Certainly you will be able to check out if other therapies might help a particular client who is not progressing, or one whose needs change. This can make it much easier for you to settle into your new role.

There will be administrative support

The clinic will have a receptionist, and perhaps also someone who can do some typing for you. The rooms will be kept clean and tidy. Someone else will order the lavatory paper and tidy up the magazines. This, of course, is what you pay for, but the payment also buys you some freedom of mind. You don't have to think about these things – and that cuts down the juggling act.

You can easily refer clients on, and receive referrals from your colleagues

Developing a list of effective colleagues in other disciplines is part of becoming a good professional. Often a client may need more than one kind of help, and one can feel that another therapy would usefully support or complement what we are doing for our client. Sometimes we feel that we have reached the limits of what we can do, but that the client could usefully shift the focus of their work in another direction or to another aspect of the problem. For example, a child who had received homoeopathic help for allergies was referred by her homoeopath to an osteopath working in the same clinic because he felt that part of her problem might be mechanical – it turned out to be a traumatic holding in the back, dating to a fall at gym that occurred long ago.

Over time, it is a good idea to build up a personal list of practitioners in other disciplines whom you feel confident to recommend, relying on personal knowledge or information from clients who have found their work helpful.

In a clinic, part of this is done for you. Make a point of finding out about what the others do, if there is no formal introduction system, so that you can cross-refer to them. Make sure they know what you do, so that they in turn can suggest your name to some of their clients. Some clinics have regular staff meetings, or even staff seminars to build up these contacts.

It is sometimes possible to discuss cases with colleagues

Obviously, if a client is passed from one practitioner to another, the two therapists will discuss the case, and may well update from time to time afterwards. But even if there has been no referring on, you are likely to be able to use informal openings to discuss a patient. This can be particularly helpful where some issue arises which is really about practice management rather than about the specifics of treatment – the kind of issue which arises in most therapies, e.g. dependency, anxiety, lateness. It can be good to know that this problem is encountered by others and doesn't just happen to you because you are newly qualified. On the other hand, experience may have led to some inventive tips and wrinkles which can save you reinventing the wheel.

It is easier to leave work behind

We have talked about this earlier, from the viewpoint of working at home. It can be really helpful to role and boundary management to go somewhere different to work, and to leave work to become a private person again. Taking off your working coat or personal uniform, tidying up and closing the door of your therapy room are good symbolic gestures and makers of these transitions.

You may be able to share advertising and publicity

The clinic will have a listed phone number and may be in the Yellow Pages (in our experience, a source of about one-third of referrals). Even if you advertise yourself individually, this will expand your public profile. Clients seeking help may find the clinic first, if they are not sure what therapy will help them or if they don't have the name of a particular therapist from a friend or doctor's recommendation. The reputation of the clinic is important here, and in assessing whether to take a room in a particular clinic, try to find out its local reputation and how long it has been in business. If a clinic is new, it may still be a good one, as often new clinics are formed when one or more practitioners – who may have been established a long time – move on and take the bulk of their clients with them. In this case, the clinic builds its reputation on those of its established practitioners rather than the other way around. Either will benefit you as a new practitioner.

Disadvantages

You won't be making the initial phone contact

We devoted a whole chapter (Ch. 3) to the importance of this first contact situation, so clearly we believe that it can be very important in aiding a good working match between client and therapist. If you work in a clinic, that vetting and reading between the lines will be out of your hands. Naturally, good receptionists have plenty of experience and may well pass on to you their impressions of clients who stand out in one way or another. But they will also be making bookings for a number of other therapists, with payments to collect and bookings to arrange for follow-up or ongoing appointments, as well as answering the phone, so it would be fair to say that you would only get a fraction of the information from them that you would gather for yourself.

They will have their own ways of dealing with clients – certainly not involving a 10 minute exploratory conversation with each person who phones in! You may be able to brief your receptionist on the kinds of information you feel are essential to you, and you will need to rely more on information leaflets to inform the client about you. This in turn may cost you more, since you may find you need to send out a leaflet to everyone who enquires about your therapy to cover the kind of tailor-made answers you would give if you were speaking to them yourself.

A receptionist won't sieve clients for you

Even though an experienced receptionist has access to just the same wealth of unconscious skill in assessing people as you are calling on, they won't be able to sort out 'good' and difficult or 'dodgy' clients for you. This may mean that some get through to you whom you would have found ways to avoid taking on if you yourself had talked with them. Again, you can tell the receptionist to trust their own judgement if they feel doubtful – to say, for example, that you are rather booked up and that they will have to check your availability before going ahead with an appointment. But even if the receptionist is willing to take on this extra responsibility, neither of you can be entirely sure that their judgement is close enough to yours.

You may have to pay for unbooked time

Clinics usually contract with therapists on the basis of whole or half-day sessions. It can be very galling to know that your fixed costs are having to be paid even if you are a client or two short – your earnings after cost get eroded and you are effectively paying out for nothing. In addition, as we have said before, it can be annoying to have to fill in a gap between clients. You may have notes to make or a book to read, but there can sometimes be a strong sense that this is just filling in time.

You don't keep all you earn

Clearly, you are getting quite substantial facilities in return for your payment to the clinic, but therapists can begrudge handing over some of their hard-won earnings – particularly as you get better known and begin to feel you are attracting clients on your own merit and through personal recommendations. This may be the time to consider a move to your own premises.

Travelling out to work can take time and may involve hassle

This is the obverse of the flexibility of working at home. You have to go out to work, which involves travelling time and travelling expense. (One therapist we know found that when she and her husband decided to give up their second car it took her 1.5 hours by public transport to get to her workplace, as against 20 minutes and minimal petrol on the days when she had the use of the car.) Even if you drive, traffic jams, weather conditions and congested parking can all affect you.

There is less flexibility

In addition to gaps in your schedule, you are constrained by your arrangement with the clinic to work on the days you have booked. This can lend structure to your life, but can make it difficult to accommodate personal needs, treats or priorities like the school outing, birthdays or childhood illnesses.

It is less easy to personalise your setting

We talked in the very first chapter about a friend's off-putting experience in a bare, undecorated room at her doctor's surgery. Many clinics are attractive, but even where they have been made pleasant with pictures, plants and nice soft furnishings, the taste isn't necessarily your taste. If you are only renting for some sessions, your room will be used by other therapists and may well communicate an anonymity to your clients. Chapter 11 on personal style discusses relatively simple ways to personalise your room while you are in it, but inevitably this will involve ferrying some of your personal accessories in with you – easier in summer, but what about wet winter days when you don't have enough hands for your portable files, your oil burner, your charts and your umbrella?

A clinic can seem cold or impersonal to clients

Some clients may find seeing a therapist in a clinic quite impersonal and reminiscent of doctors' surgeries – even the magazines may be as dog-eared or old, and the sight of other patients waiting just as reinforcing of distress or physical vulnerability. Timid and anxious patients are likely to be particularly put off. If they have already trudged around from doctor to specialist to hospital for some intractable or so-called psychosomatic complaint, this can get things off to a poor start.

Equipment may not be exactly what you want

We all rely heavily on our equipment – it is not 'only' a couch, but something whose height and adjustability suit us more or less exactly and can make our work that much easier. Where the equipment belongs to the clinic and is used by several people, maintenance becomes more of an issue and you can't keep such a close eye on wear and tear and impending need for repairs as if you were the sole user. You may well have to take your client files in with you. We remember a busy homoeopath carting two large metal file boxes in and out, which necessitated two trips to his car on arrival and departure – not a lot, but multiply that by a number of days each week, weeks a month, and months a year...

We talked earlier about a 'clean' environment. If you are an osteopath, or a kineseologist, how do you feel about going into a room where the previous therapist has been burning essential oils? Might be very nice sometimes, but not necessarily appropriate for either you or your client who has come for a different therapy.

Clinics are businesses

In agreeing to rent a room to work in, you are making a contract with the owner or proprietor. However friendly they are, and even if they are a working therapist, they will legitimately regard the running of their clinic as a business. Some will run it efficiently, others less so. Some will be easy to deal with and fair in their contract; others may ensure that in any dispute or ambiguity they never end up as the loser. New therapists may find themselves having to accommodate therapists who have worked in the clinic longer, and through lack of experience could find themselves disadvantaged.

It is worth reading over your contract carefully before signing, and if necessary asking someone you trust – even a lawyer – to look it over for you to ensure you have as fair a deal as possible. For example, how much notice do you have to give of any holidays? Do you have to pay the full rental for that time, or a reduced rate? What does the rental of the room actually include? Find out about lighting and heating, outgoing phone calls, building insurance, use of washing machine etc. Are these included, or are they extras? Ask to see the fire regulations and/or certificate. You will still need your own personal professional indemnity insurance to work from the clinic. Find out who does reception duty when the receptionist is away or in the evenings (we have known clinics where the therapists had to take turns to fill in!).

As before, in itemising possible snags, we are not arguing that you should not work in a clinic, but only that you need to think through the various features of the setting and the organisation so that you can be sure that it is the best workplace for you. This involves working out your personal priorities.

When you go to look at a clinic, remember that you are finding out if the clinic is a good enough place for *you* to work in, not the other way around.

Working in the client's home

Advantages

You can treat clients who are unable to come to visit you

These will be clients who either lack transport or time (no car, small kids) or who are physically unable to travel. People with long-term debilitating illnesses such as MS, stroke victims and those with terminal illness may benefit enormously from your therapy. Going to them means they don't have the added stress of travel, even if they could physically manage it, and that you are not depleting their already limited energy.

You don't have to set aside space in your home

New therapists may not have an extra room in their flat/house, or for other reasons find their home unsuitable for seeing people (e.g. an invalid parent or partner, young children, living deep in the country). You might, like one of our students, be planning to move to another area of the country in a short time, and therefore be unwilling to undertake the rearrangement and the expense of converting a room even if you have one available.

It is very flexible

You can fit in with the client's needs and availability because you are not impinging on the events and lives of people you live with. You can arrange times that suit the client.

Disadvantages

You have to spend time travelling

Quite a lot of time may be taken up in travelling, particularly if you live in London, another large city or, conversely, in the depths of the country. It may be difficult to rationalise your week so as to bunch your clients, visiting those in the same area on the same day, even though this would suit you better. Even if you can, you may have to plan to have lunch out somewhere – another expense – or to take sandwiches, which can make for delightful picnics in summer but is less fun in winter.

You will have to carry equipment about

Even portable couches are quite heavy and you need to consider how practicable it will be to take one up flights of stairs to someone in a flat. It can be heavy and hard work, particularly since you will almost certainly have to make a second journey for the rest of your equipment. Doing this regularly as your caseload builds up can be tiring.

The client may be distracted by domestic interruptions

The client has as many potential distractions at home as you do, but often without the protection of an answerphone! This can impinge seriously upon some therapies.

Mums with small children may be tempted to think they can fit in a massage, for example, while older children mind the little ones, but what if a fight or another sort of emergency occurs?

Driving may be tiring

A travelling therapist, like a travelling salesman, may become stressed not by the job but by the distances and by road conditions.

You may not be able to charge enough realistically to cover your time and costs

This can be very important in your pricing. Your client may well be prepared to pay money towards your petrol, but if you are building even part of your practice around home visits you need to look very realistically at what it actually costs you to do it. If your charge for a session at your home is, say, £25, how much extra will you need to charge to earn the same rate if visiting a client 20 minutes' drive away? An extra 40 minutes (minimum) is involved. Can you charge that time at your working rate? That effectively makes the treatment quite expensive, particularly when petrol is added. If you feel you need to charge less for travelling time (not exactly therapeutic for the client) you may feel aggrieved, because after all it is still your time that is being used up. What happens when you get busier and find that for every client you see at home you are effectively earning less than for every client you see at your home or in a clinic? Does that have an adverse effect on your attitude towards home-based clients? Be honest with yourself in assessing this.

It is our experience that therapists starting up, in the first flush of enthusiasm for their therapy and for helping people in need, rarely do the maths of the exercise and cost their time and effort realistically. Our argument, as always, is that you are free to give your time for little or nothing if you choose, but that it doesn't benefit you or the client if you feel subtly exploited, however unintentionally, in working with them.

Constant change and adaptation itself contributes to stress

An on-the-hoof therapy will drain you, just as cattle driven long distances lose weight through constant movement and the stress of continual adaptation to a changing environment. You may want to think of home visits as a short-term, or emergency, way of working, since, as we have said before, maintaining you is your first priority. A tired, harassed or hassled therapist is a less effective – and before long an unwell – therapist.

Assessing the right environment

We have discussed the advantages and disadvantages of the three major settings in which most bodywork therapists are likely to work. Hospital and hospice work share some features of the clinic setting, although contract issues, emotional factors and some managerial features will be different.

We can identify a number of needs to look out for. Client and therapist share needs for:

◆ privacy

◆ (relative) quiet

◆ appropriate, adjustable light and heat

◆ easy access to needed facilities and equipment

◆ water/refreshment.

Therapists also need:

◆ secure filing methods and space

◆ storage for essential equipment

◆ additional therapeutic adjuncts or accessories (e.g. music system, facilities for washing towels).

Clients need:

◆ somewhere to wait

◆ somewhere to change/undress

◆ magazines to read while waiting

◆ parking.

In this chapter, we have considered a range of considerations beginning therapists need to bear in mind when choosing their workplace. In assessing these, your needs and preferences as a person are of paramount importance. If you are at ease in your environment, this will go a long way towards helping you create a good atmosphere for your therapy. It will even offset some disadvantages, or help you minimise their effect on the client. The American business guru, Tom Peters, quotes a firm whose slogan was: 'Remember, the customer always comes second.' It is, he emphasises, the work force which comes first.

In this case, *you* are your work force. *You* have to come first so that you can give of your best to your clients. Each client will see you, at most, once a week and often at longer intervals. You will be seeing your clients anything up to 4 or 5 days a week, so your workplace (or places) must suit you, cause you minimal inconvenience or stress. It is our belief, and our experience, that making the right choice *for you* will allow you to offer yourself and your skills with greatest ease and freedom to those who seek your help.

11 Your style

In this chapter, we will explore all the issues of making your practice uniquely yours. In other words, we will look at how you stamp your own personal style on your professional practice. We will explore such issues as organising and designing your stationery, style and content of your treatment room, colour schemes, clothing etc.

It is important for therapists to remember that people interpret what they perceive, and act on this perception. The down-side of this is that often the messages received are not always what was intended, and not necessarily the reality. To help cut back on possible misinterpretation, therapists need to carry a constant awareness of what can influence perception.

It is also important to remember that your client will have engaged in a process of preparation and anticipation before they enter your treatment room, and you want to be able to influence this process positively by your use of stationery, answerphone messages etc., and by your professional style.

Stationery

Once you have decided to set up a practice the real hard work begins! Whether you choose to practise from home or from a clinic (or indeed both), you will still need to think about stationery, but even before that you have to give thought to what you are going to be called. If you are lucky enough to have your own set of treatment rooms separate from your home then you may want to give thought to a title that involves:

◆ your brand of therapy

◆ the word 'practice'

◆ your name.

Taking these three issues means that you can use any combination, e.g. 'Jane Green's aromatherapy practice'; 'John H Smith Chiropractor'; 'John H Smith Chiropractic Clinic'; 'J H Green Aromatherapy Treatment Centre'; 'J H Green Sports Injuries and Massage Clinic'.

Practising from home may mean that you just want to use your name and your chosen practice, e.g. 'L Powell Aromatherapist'; 'G Slade Chiropractor'; 'L Douglas Physiotherapist'.

Whatever you finally decide, our suggestion is that you keep your 'title' simple and as clear as possible; that way it will be more easily remembered!

Having decided on what you want to be called, now you can think about designing your stationery. In Chapter 2, we talked about advertising and also your target client group. In particular, we asked you to think about the preferences you had in relation to your clients with a view to advertising. Now we ask you to think about your target client group again, only this time with a view to designing your stationery and, in particular, the colour of your stationery.

> Before we do this, we suggest that you carry out a very simple exercise which will help to demonstrate the points that follow. Take out all the various business cards that you have in your wallet, briefcase etc. (if you don't have any to hand, borrow some from somebody else). Spread them out in front of you and see if you can draw any meaning or inference from the design and colour that is before you. Forget for the moment the amount of writing on the cards but pay special attention to the design and colour used.

The kinds of things that you might notice are the impact of black on white, and the kinds of professions that use this, i.e. consultants, bankers, accountants, people who want to note a high degree of professionalism (that does not mean that colour is not professional). Other 'professional' cards are normally single colour ink on single colour paper. It can certainly be argued that such a colour combination is quite stark and quite cold, and indeed if you think about professions that we have just talked about, this may be because they don't feel there is much warmth 'in what they do'! What we are asking you to think about is the kind of impression that these colour combinations leave you with as a recipient. For instance, if you were handed a business card of an accountant that displayed in the right-hand corner a rainbow and underneath the phrase,

'Helping to put you in touch with your crock of gold', you may find this amusing and think this is just the accountant for you. However, other people might find such a business card too flippant and be totally put off by it.

Your design needs to be targeted to the type of audience that you want to reach. If you want your client group to come from professional business people, keep your stationery clear and simple (it also means that you will cut down on the expense – the more colour you use, the more expensive it becomes).

Take time to design your stationery. Take time to think about what the colour of any logo that you use actually denotes. Go away and do your research, collect other people's stationery: what do you like or dislike about the design and the colour; what does it 'say' to you? Take, for instance, the 'Body Shop', a clear title that could not be misconstrued by anybody. When Anita Roddick first started, people knew from her title and her logo what they would find in her shop – anything and everything to do with the body.

Having got a design that you feel comfortable with, which you believe denotes your style and the type of practice that you wish to promote, pass it around to friends and acquaintances and perhaps to old colleagues, and ask them to be honest in their opinion. Ask them: 'How do you feel about this, what does this say to you? Would you be interested in going to this person for a treatment? If so, why? If you could improve this design or layout what would you change, and why?'

It is at this stage that other people's opinions are going to be important to you. Remember you are inviting honest criticism of a design, not of your practice. Therefore welcome this criticism and take on board their comments. After all, it's up to you whether you do anything about them; this is your stationery and your style.

The problem with this kind of project is that often we can become too close; we are too aware of what we are involved in, and less aware of the impact that words and colour can have on other people. Remember that communication takes place in the mind of the other: you know what you mean by your notepaper, your title and your logo but you don't know at this stage how it will be received by other people. So check it out. Hand it around to as many people as possible and invite their honest criticism.

If you want a clear 'professional' statement about who you are and what you do, you may well choose black on white, blue, or grey etc. (We have heard some people say that grey is boring; others find it very restful. It depends on who, i.e. what type of person, is receiving it.)

Green is becoming a very popular colour with a good many 'holistic' therapists. Do remember to check all of these colours in both daylight and artificial light. What to you is a gentle shade of green could well remind others of their last channel crossing!

When thinking about colour and design, it will pay you to consult your local printer or art designer – cost permitting. Not only are they the experts in colour and design, but they can advise you on colour combinations and layout and show you designs that others have used.

If money is tight, or stationery is not one of your top priority outlays, then you may want to consider a two stage process, the first part of which you could do yourself on a local printing machine (found on most large railway stations and larger stationery shops, and very effective they are too). This would be black on white, and you can experiment with type face and design for quite a small cost. Another advantage of this route is that you can live with the design for a while before making your final decision. The second phase could be to refine your design and type face, and maybe add colour.

Whichever route you decide to go, remember a few basic rules:

◆ Who is the stationery designed to be received by?

◆ What do you want it to reflect about your practice and your professionalism?

◆ How is it likely to be received by others? Make sure the layout is clear

◆ Check it out! Show your draft designs to others and invite criticism

◆ Go for the best that you can afford

◆ Don't stop until you are 100% satisfied.

The other factor to consider, of course, is that if you choose a route that involves black and one other colour on your paper then 'plates' will need to be made and this initial outlay can be expensive and even more costly to change.

Why have we suggested that you go for the best that you can afford? It's quite simple – your stationery and advertising material (which will carry your name and details) need to 'travel' well. The higher the quality of paper that you use, the crisper it will be on arrival – regardless of post and handling – and the more professional it will look.

Having decided on your design and colour scheme, now you have to decide what you want, e.g. note paper, compliments slips, business cards. You also need to decide on size and quantity. Let us deal with size first. The sizing commonly used for standard professional note paper is A4; another smaller size that can be used is A5.

When considering the size, once again give thought to what you will use the paper for, and the type of practice that you are looking to establish. If your intention is to lecture/teach/train as well as having individual clients, in the first instance your note paper may well need to double as invoices and therefore the A5 size could be the most efficient. If you are not yet ready to produce a specific flier, i.e. you are just starting, the A4 will provide you with ample space to give a brief description of who you are and the type of practice you are running. If, however, you want to use your note paper more as a 'Dear Miss Smith, Thank you for your enquiry... I have pleasure in enclosing details... etc.' then you may feel that the smaller A5 size is for you.

The above example also serves to illustrate the use of a compliments slip. Compliments slips these days usually accompany the main point of the correspondence, e.g. a package, goods in transit, books etc. which require very little, if any, other written explanation. Quite a few people use compliments slips instead of a letter, e.g. 'Dear Miss Smith, Thank you for your call. This is to confirm your appointment on...'.

Generally, compliments slips are normally 210 mm × 145 mm in size and will be identical in design and layout to your stationery and business cards.

Another use for the compliments slip is to use either the front or the reverse as an appointment card.

And so to the continuing debate amongst bodywork therapists about the need for business cards. Our experience has shown that the majority of chiropractors, acupuncturists, osteopaths, physiotherapists and sports massage practitioners are in favour of business cards whilst some aromatherapists, reflexologists, beauty therapists etc. are still not 100% sure whether the business card route is one that they want to follow.

Obviously you need to decide for yourself whether business cards are a useful way of you spending your money. One of the wonderful things about business cards is that they also 'travel well'. They can be carried in large quantities without too much effort and handed out very easily to people. It is common practice for a business card to be the same size as a credit card, i.e. 85 mm × 55 mm.

It is becoming more common amongst bodywork therapists to use the business card as an appointment card as well, i.e. the front of the card carries the name of the practitioner and the back carries an appointment date and time. This seems to be a very economical, useful and business-orientated practice.

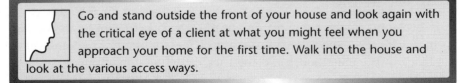

We would like you to take a few minutes to think about business cards; whether you like the idea or dislike the idea, and what has contributed to your feeling. Having noted these points down, if you find that you have a bias against business cards, give some thought to how you could make them work for you and your practice. If you find yourself in favour of business cards, think about how you could make even greater use of them in a way that is uniquely yours.

Treatment rooms

Let us now look at how you can create your individual style in your treatment room. As we have discussed in previous chapters, there are four places from which you can practise:

◆ your home – with a dedicated treatment room

◆ a room in your home that you use for other purposes as well as therapy

◆ a treatment room in a clinic

◆ a room in the client's home.

A dedicated treatment room in your home.

This is perhaps the easiest of all the options you have in terms of stamping your style and personality. But, having said that, you also have to remember that in the majority of cases, to reach your treatment room your clients will have to walk through your house. It will therefore be important that all access ways are kept clean and tidy, and you may perhaps find it useful to think again about the impression that the front of your house and the access ways to your treatment room give to other people.

Go and stand outside the front of your house and look again with the critical eye of a client at what you might feel when you approach your home for the first time. Walk into the house and look at the various access ways.

As a client, what might you notice that might impress you, or leave you less than happy? Note all these points and put them into debit and credit columns. On the credit side, you might wish to note clean and tidy garden, welcoming front door, sparkling windows, nice aspect; on the debit side, you might note that paintwork needs repair, curtains look untidy and dishevelled from the outside. Internally, on the credit side – attractive pictures, good paintwork; on the debit side – fraying carpet.

Now, we are not suggesting that in order to start your own practice from home you have to organise a major DIY face-lift on your house. Very few of us are in a position to do that, especially when we are starting our own business. What we are suggesting, however, is that, having identified positive features about both the outside and inside of your home, highlighting these features or putting more emphasis on them will take attention away from things that you intend to improve at a later date.

Look again at the debit and credit list that you have made. Could it be that a few strategically placed flowers would draw a person's eye to the garden rather than anywhere else? Making sure windows are always kept in sparkling condition could soon become a feature that people remember about your home. Moving on to the inside, if you have attractive pictures on the wall then perhaps more pictures, or subtle lighting to enhance the ones that you already have, will take people's eye. There are many ways – many of them inexpensive – that you can re-work the outside and the inside of your home so that they communicate to your clients your style and your professionalism.

We have talked before about the fact that your treatment room needs to offer privacy, and that it needs to be warm and comfortable, but it also needs to denote your style of practice. So do think carefully about the kind of treatment room that you want, the kind of room that you want to practise in, a room that will allow you to work as well as offering comfort and relaxation to your clients.

Do you want a clean clinical treatment room with very few personal effects? Will your treatment room also contain all your working materials, e.g. books, charts etc.? If so, how and where will you store them, and what kind of colour scheme do you feel will match the mood and task of the room? Do you want, through colour and style, to have a warm, welcoming, relaxing treatment room with very little working material around, i.e. warm colours on the wall, flowers, a small changing area and your treatment couch as the centre and pivotal piece of furniture? We could go on and turn this book into a design module for treatment rooms but that is not our intention! Whatever type of treatment room you decide on – as with your stationery – give plenty of thought to how it will appear to other people: ask advice, look through design books and magazines, and gather ideas that you can turn into your own.

If, when you start designing your room, money is a key consideration, then you may want to think about going for new paintwork and using the paintwork, i.e. the colour and natural light, to create an effect for you. By keeping your room clean and simple, you can often change its appearance with the addition of pictures or prints and even a vase of flowers. If you are fortunate to have a room with large windows but are not yet in a position to curtain them, or a large room that initially affords too much space, you could think about going to pine shops or 'trash and treasure' shops, and investing in some pine, cane or hardwood folding screens. These screens can either be put up and used in their natural state or material or even pictures can be placed on them. They could then cover a corner, conceal a window and would be an interesting and exciting way of stamping your style. Think about the things that bring joy to you – are they suitable for your treatment room, e.g. plants, flowers, use of colour, materials, books, music? The list is endless.

> Take a few moments to jot down how you could transform a room into a treatment room that would be professional and yet demonstrate your style. In other words, it would be *your* treatment room. Before you know it, and with a little imagination, you could be in demand designing treatment rooms!

Non-dedicated treatment room in your own home

A good many therapists who are in the process of developing their practice from home start with a dual-purpose room. It has to be said, however, that this is the least feasible option and is best avoided if at all possible, as it is a room that will need both careful planning and probably disguising! Having said this, we do acknowledge that for some therapists it is their only option.

Things to remember when trying to decide which room is best suited to the dual function are:

◆ where it is situated in the house, i.e. ease of access

◆ its position in relation to the bathroom and the kitchen (why is it that the noxious smells linger longer than any others?)

◆ how much non-treatment use it will have, i.e. how much 'clearing' you will have to do each time you use it

◆ size and (very important) warmth.

No matter which room you use, you will need to give careful thought to light. The use of small or free-standing lamps can create the illusion of warmth and therapeutic space, and can be put in place quite quickly. Do your personal belongings contribute to, or detract from, the therapeutic atmosphere, and how quickly and safely can they be moved? Where can clothes be hung?

Dining room

Make sure that you have enough room to create the illusion of space. If you do not need to move the dining room table, then do cover it, and change its use so that it becomes an integral part of your treatment room, e.g. cover with a throw, use for oils, towels, diary, notes, therapy reference books etc.

Sitting room

As with the dining room, space is a vital factor. If you have a large room, then move the furniture to create a distinct 'sitting' area and open the rest as your treatment room. If it is not a large room, then move as much of the furniture as possible in order to create the space inside the sitting area. The clever use of throws can change the shape and design of furniture, and again means that its function can be changed.

Do remember to clear away newspapers, magazines etc., and either turn on the answerphone or, if you haven't got one, turn off the ringer on the telephone.

Think about the position of your windows in relation to privacy and also light. A south-facing room is wonderful, but not if it means that the light is shining into either your face or that of your client.

Conservatory

With this kind of space, windows, privacy and warmth are very high on the agenda. The use of rugs and folding panels can help to build a feeling of warmth and professional intimacy. If you have lots of plants in the conservatory, think about how they will affect your clients. If you are not sure, then moving them is better than helping to bring on an allergy attack!

Spare bedrooms

The spare bedroom is probably one of the best rooms to use. A throw over the bed with some matching cushions immediately changes its use, provides a storage area and gives you and your client a place to sit. If there is a dressing table or chest of drawers in the room, either cover it with a matching throw and use for diary and notes, or, if that is not possible, then do clear away all personal belongings. If it really is a 'spare room' then you will probably be able to keep charts and books etc. in it full time and decorate it in a way that allows it to move effortlessly from one function to another.

Own bedroom

This, we suggest, is the final option, but if it has to be used then decorate in a neutral colour, and when it is being used as a treatment room, cover the bed with a throw that, if possible, matches your curtains and cushions. Do try to create as much of an 'unbedroomy' atmosphere as possible, with personal belongings put away and clever use of charts, books etc.

A way of creating the illusion of space is to try and colour-coordinate, as much as possible, throws, cushions, towels, gowns, etc. It also adds to the transformation. It will be in your choice of colourings that you will create your own distinctive style.

A treatment room in a clinic

The ease or difficulty with which you stamp your style on a room in a clinic will be governed in part by whether you have exclusive use of the room and any conditions regarding decor set by the clinic owners.

If you have exclusive use of the room then the issues we discussed in a dedicated treatment room will apply. If you rent the room on either a daily or part time basis, then some of the extra considerations you might have are such things as how much time you have available to 'set up' the room, what it already contains that may need improving or disguising, whether there is storage space available or whether you have to bring all these extras in every time. (If you can think of others, do jot them down, so that if and when you rent clinic space you have them available for discussion *and* negotiation.) All of these issues will inform just how much of your own style you can imprint on the room.

Working from the client's home

It is worth making some preliminary enquiries as to *which room* you will be able to use, and how much space is available, *before* you confirm the booking. It will avoid all sorts of horrors and time problems on the day of treatment. It allows you to check out such issues as privacy, possible interruptions, etc. It also gives the client time to make alternative arrangements concerning incoming telephone calls, children/family members returning home or remaining in the house, and other such issues.

In consultation with your client, you will need to decide how appropriate or necessary it is to move furniture and, if curtains need to be closed for privacy, what other forms of lighting are available.

Another useful check is availability of car parking, and *how close it is* to the client's house! (We will let your imagination create that picture!)

On arrival, be clear about what you want your client to do or not do. For instance, is it appropriate for them to help you with setting up your equipment, or would you rather they sat and relaxed? If they do sit quietly, it may be better that they do it in another room – space permitting – to allow you the time and space to organise yourself and 'create' your working area.

It may well be that your unique style manifests itself in giving your clients breathing or visualising exercises to carry out whilst you are setting up, or in the harmonising colours of the towels you use.

Mode of dress

To uniform or not to uniform, that is the perennial question. Most therapists these days prefer to wear some kind of clothing that denotes uniform, i.e. 'official or standard dress' (*Collins Dictionary* definition), which is comfortable.

If you are not happy with the idea of a 'uniform', think about how a uniform could be perceived by the client within your particular therapy. Most people with whom we have discussed this see a uniform as supportive, marking a clear division between the person and the professional: ' I felt more comfortable removing my clothes... Their uniform was their professional badge.' A few felt that a uniform was too clinical and distanced them from the therapist.

One of our clients recounted how it had been agreed that she could have a Saturday morning appointment with her osteopath who didn't normally see clients at the weekend. On arrival at the clinic, she was met by her osteopath who was full of profuse apologies for not wearing a white coat; one had been washed and was not yet dry, and the other needed washing. Our client stated that she felt extremely uncomfortable removing her clothing because 'he didn't look like my osteopath any more, but like any other chap'.

Wearing a uniform doesn't necessarily mean a white coat. If you find the idea of a white coat too formal, you could think about a white T-shirt/sweatshirt with white slacks, or you could opt for a coat in a pale or cream colour.

 Experiment by taking soundings from people around you. How would they react to your various ideas and colour schemes if they were your clients?

Here are some advantages of a uniform:

◆ it saves on other clothes

◆ if working from home, it helps to get into, and out of, role and helps the therapist to make the transition

◆ most people see a uniform as supportive

◆ a white uniform is often seen as being aligned to some form of medical model, and therefore as professional.

It will be up to you to make the decision – whatever you wear has to look clean, presentable and be of a colour and design that is congruent with your therapy.

In ending this chapter on style, we would ask you to bear in mind that everything communicates something to someone. Therefore, be aware of what clothing, hair, make-up, aftershave and condition of hands and nails *could* communicate to your client. If your hair is long, it will need to be tied back; jewellery and make-up should be discreet; don't wear overpowering perfume or aftershave; and hands and nails should be scrupulously clean.

Do dress to be comfortable, but most importantly of all, dress as a professional.

12 Managing personal involvement

In this chapter, we shall be looking at four main potential areas of difficulty in managing your personal interaction with a client:

◆ becoming emotionally too close to the client (over-involved)

◆ dependence issues

◆ transference and counter-transference

◆ sexual issues.

We will use examples to illustrate some of the ways therapists may encounter these problems in practice, since they are mostly quite subtle and rarely grossly obvious, and suggest steps that can be taken to restore a more professional pattern of interaction.

We said at the very beginning of the book that it is our belief that what we offer to the client in our interaction goes beyond our learned therapeutic skills and includes much of ourselves, both in terms that we would recognise and in much subtler ways that rest upon our life experience. We meet the client as a person with a helping intent. Bodywork, too, is a close and personal form of work, and caring touch makes a bridge between us. Many clients will visit us in some form of physical or emotional discomfort, pain or distress, which inevitably call forth responses from us. We will be involved in the healing and creative use of this personal link with our clients.

As therapists, it is our responsibility to monitor this interaction and to ensure, as best we can, that it is beneficial to the client. We think and feel as the individuals we are, but we are in a role relationship where the expression of our thoughts and feelings is constrained within professional, not personal, limits.

The client, of course, comes with their own attitudes, values, expectations, learned behaviour patterns and hopes, quite apart from the vulnerability of their immediate need. They may project unreasonable hopes or expectations onto us, or may cast us into role partnerships familiar to them from their previous experience. Sometimes we may fall into these quite neatly and automatically, but at other times there may be an obvious lack of fit!

All this is part of normal human interaction. Being aware of what is, or may be, going on helps us to use our links and time with the client wisely, protecting both them and ourselves from some of the potential hazards which can arise.

Becoming emotionally too close

If it is important to form a relationship with the client, how can the therapist know when they are 'too close'? Too close for what?

Degrees of closeness involve boundaries, which in our experience are among the most important, and helpful, factors in successful relationships. In the case of therapy, the client comes with a problem or difficulty for which they want help. In consulting a body therapist, they want help with something they experience primarily in physical ways. Maintaining a clear boundary of professionalism means that both partners in the therapy are able to focus their respective energies on working to improve that problem. If the therapist becomes 'too close', they will cease to be as fully helpful as they might be.

Let's take some examples. The client may already have visited several different kinds of helper, without success. They may feel helpless and despondent. An empathic therapist will connect with these feelings – being human, we have all felt similar things. This allows us to respond sensitively and avoid being too bracing or dismissive of the client's fears. But if we dig too deeply into our own memories of helplessness, which may be stimulated by the client's plight, by our liking of them as a person or by the depth and painfulness of similar experiences we have had in the past, we can end up feeling just as helpless as they do. We may find ourselves thinking, 'How can I as an inexperienced therapist possibly succeed where others have failed?' or 'I don't think I know enough to help this person', or even 'I wonder if this is a hopeless case after all?'

In this case, our overidentification with the client has effectively made us less helpful to them, although it stemmed from the very best motives and the most sensitive response. We would have been more helpful if we had been able to remind ourselves that of course the client's helplessness *would* be great, since their previous treatment had not helped, and then asked ourselves honestly if we really believed ours would be significantly different. The self-talk might then have been more positive and less emotional, and the response to the client would have provided a clear sense of emotional support (what social workers and psychologists sometimes call 'holding') which rested on knowledge and professionalism.

Another closeness/boundary issue can arise when the therapist and client find each other very likeable. Naturally, mutual liking can make therapy a very pleasant and rewarding experience for both parties, but it too can threaten the client's feelings of professional and impartial support and safety. Apart from obvious fudging of professional boundaries like dating clients, there are many more subtle violations of the professional distance between client and therapist.

Telling the client things about your life, thoughts and feelings may indicate that the relationship is moving towards a friendship and that the therapeutic focus is being lost. The client may value this move just as much as the therapist, but it is still an inadvisable shift in therapeutic terms. We will look at issues of sexual attraction later in the chapter, but some of the same issues are raised by less acute feelings developing between client and therapist.

Signs and symptoms of blurred or lost focus are:

◆ when you worry about the client

◆ when you think frequently about the client

◆ when you find yourself fantasising about them

◆ when personal material or issues intrude into the treatment

◆ when you look forward to appointments with that client (or dread them).

We suggest that, if you become aware of any of these responses in yourself, you make time to think through how you feel and to review how the interaction between you and the client has led up to this. Good options at this point are to:

◆ write down anything that seems relevant

◆ talk through the issues in supervision, if you receive it, or with a colleague or friend whom you can trust to be impartial (and if necessary to confront you honestly, as well as reassuring you if appropriate)

◆ ask yourself if the proper boundaries can be gently restored by modifying your own behaviour without discussing things with the client

◆ consider whether you should talk openly with the client

◆ consider whether you should refer the client to another therapist, and in this case ask yourself how you would like the relationship with the client to be maintained.

While the more insidious problems occur where client and therapist like each other, similar boundary issues can occur where the therapist feels an irritation or dislike for the client, and again it is much better to address the issue than to soldier on with the risk of giving the client less than they have a right to expect. Another therapist might find it easier to work with them, or might even like them.

While we have a responsibility to work at our best with our clients, it is important to remember that we do not need to work with every potential client and that passing them on may give them, and another therapist, a chance of a better working relationship, and better help, than they could have with us.

Consider the following scenarios:

◆ You go to a party given by a therapist colleague, who introduces you to a number of people, among them three or four whom she introduces as 'one of my clients'. Clearly, they seem on friendly terms with her. One asks you if you know if the colleague's sister has recovered from flu yet. Another comments on a film they recently saw together. A third indicates in conversation that she is currently having therapy with your colleague.

◆ Two clients phone you within half-an-hour of each other to cancel appointments for the next day. You are rather irritated, although both have understandable reasons and accept that they will have to pay you an agreed cancellation fee. However, you realise as you make plans to rearrange your day that you are more disappointed not to be seeing one of them than the other.

◆ You wake in the night having had a very vivid dream about a client, in which you have been searching for them in a large shopping mall, becoming increasingly anxious that some accident may have befallen them.

◆ You are having a meal at a favourite restaurant with a friend/partner when a familiar voice calls your name. You look round and see one of your clients in the midst of a large group of people apparently celebrating something. Your client asks if you and your partner would like to join them.

Each scenario could well occur. Take a little while to sort out what issues you think might be involved. What kind of response would help to keep professional boundaries in place, while respecting both the client and yourself? In particular, how does being professional while on duty differ from being professional when off duty? How might you respond at the time, and would you need/wish to follow up that response in any way when in your professional setting? There are no tidy right answers, only right principles!

Dealing with dependence issues

When we visit a professional, we are all in a potentially dependent position because of our difficulty and their assumed expertise. Even in our initial contact with them (see Ch. 3), we may be signalling that we hope to be cured or rescued. For most of us, visits to doctors over the years have reinforced this. We might call this a situational dependency (i.e. the situation creates or fosters it). While recognising that even at the very outset it is usually helpful to indicate to clients that they are partners in getting better, rather than passive receivers of our therapy, we do also need to train ourselves to spot clients who bring a more personal or rooted dependency into their treatment with us.

Signs of dependency

Signs of dependency are when a client:

◆ exhibits 'tell me what to do next' behaviour

◆ asks frequent questions which require an 'expert' response

◆ routes everything through to you for approval – how would you do it; what do you think; what would be the best way; what would you like me to do; is that right?

◆ telephones frequently to update you on their progress

◆ telephones frequently about apparent (probably not actual) emergencies

◆ asks for more frequent appointments than necessary

◆ seems reluctant to space appointments out although condition is improving.

In each of these cases, there is an overt message and an implied one. The implied messages are that you know better than the client; that they find it difficult to manage without you, or without being told what to do; that they are scared of being on their own again; and that they would like even more support.

It is reasonable to assume that the client is importing an existing need for direction and probably for emotional support into the therapy. Perhaps they have been trained by parents or partners to take a submissive role. They lack confidence in operating independently. Being unwell or in pain will have accentuated whatever dependency needs they already have, since illness and uncertainty tend to make everyone regress to earlier developmental stages or roles, however capable or independent they are.

Many therapists will feel anxious when they experience the pressure of others' dependency. They may also feel uncertain (it's hard to be viewed as an expert, particularly when we know just how limited or new our expertise really is) and perhaps irritated. Phone calls and letters carrying 'unnecessary' updates and queries can begin to make us feel as though we are being pestered, and it is very easy and natural to begin to withdraw or close down emotionally, becoming impatient.

It is important to monitor your responses and quickly to notice such changes from how you used to feel about this client or how your feelings about this client differ from those about other clients.

Suggested courses of action

◆ Ask yourself if you have inadvertently sought or encouraged dependency. A client with highly dependent needs will easily take 'normal' comments like 'You're really doing a good job in keeping up those exercises' as praise for good behaviour. We all value praise and it quickly connects us with a multiplicity of childhood situations in which teachers and parents praised us for being 'good'. This is particularly likely to happen, of course, where a client is being praised for doing their 'homework', since this task itself is reminiscent of childhood pupillage. You might also have inadvertently set yourself up as a teacher or parental figure because you are comfortable in those roles, in which case your needs and preferences will be interlocking with those of your client.

◆ Discuss the situation with your supervisor or a colleague or friend whom you can trust to give you an objective view.

◆ Reflect your observations back to the client in a gentle, hypothetical way so that they do not feel confronted or criticised. Statements which begin 'I've noticed that...', 'I wonder if...?', 'Have you also felt...?', 'It seems to me as if...' may all help to establish an atmosphere of mutual reflection and evaluation which in itself begins to shift the role relationship towards greater equality. For obvious reasons, it is particularly important not to reinforce your implied status and their dependency by interpretive or defining statements which 'tell them how it is' or which patronise them.

◆ Work towards greater client independence. Without snatching your support from under the client's feet and virtually asking them to grow up and act their age, encourage them to feel that they can take responsibility for part of their treatment, to believe that they will survive with a slightly longer gap between appointments. You can use words that imply a causal connection: '*Since* you've done your home tasks so conscientiously, you *will be able* to...'. You can point out achievements: 'Managing this holiday break so effectively tells you you're becoming more independent and able to help yourself now'. You can allow a slightly longer time between receiving a message from the client and replying to it than you think the client would like, but then encourage by saying something like: 'It was really good to get your message and know how well you've been doing'.

◆ It may also be useful to remind them, implicitly or explicitly, that you too have a private life, as well as a number of clients apart from them, and therefore make a general habit of responding to client queries and messages only during your work time. (If work time for you includes some evenings, they still need to know that on certain days or outside certain hours, you regard yourself as being off duty and don't deal with work issues. Making this as a general point allows all but the most self-obsessed clients to realise that you are not picking specifically on them to ignore!)

You arrive at your clinic to begin work and notice one of your clients in the waiting room, although you are not expecting to see them that day. You check your diary with the receptionist, who tells you that the client was waiting on the doorstep when she arrived and seems anxious. What do you do next?

A client has had a recurrence of a problem for which you treated them some time before. Although the difficulty is not serious, it is irritatingly debilitating and the client tends to panic, fearing each time that they will not get better again. You tell the client that fortnightly treatment coupled with a self-care programme is the best approach in your view, reminding them that this has helped previous acute episodes. Two days after their session with you, the client leaves several messages expressing anxiety and asking for a further, urgent appointment. How do you respond?

In addition to your work in the session, you suggest that a client undertakes a number of exercises at home and asks their partner to help them with some gentle massage. The client asks if they could see you twice weekly instead, as they are fearful of making the condition worse through amateur treatment. You know they could afford extra sessions and just at the moment your workload would allow you to fit them in. What are the pros and cons of agreeing?

Transference

While transference most commonly occurs within psychotherapy, and indeed is encouraged by some schools of psychotherapy because they believe it is fundamental to therapeutic change and growth, it does also occur within other therapies, particularly where treatment is long-term or intense. Freud coined the term to describe a process in which the client transfers into the therapeutic relationship feelings, behaviours and assumptions which were experienced within past important relationships, particularly those of family and childhood. It is as though the state of anxiety or distress, and the situational dependence of being a client visiting an expert helper, triggers patterns formed long ago in other dependent relationships, usually with parents and family members. Because of the therapist's status as expert, the client is particularly acutely aware of many details which ostensibly have nothing to do with the substance of the therapy. This is an entirely normal reaction: when we meet a new, high-status person we notice clothing, tone of voice, verbal and body language, and when we are anxious or confused we hang on to even casual statements with particular attentiveness.

However, this means that as therapists we need to be particularly aware of two things: first, that as far as the client is concerned our words and actions are not casual or incidental; and second, that the way the client responds to us may have more to do with the baggage they bring with them than with the here and now.

It is easier, of course, to spot transference behaviour when what is said or done is clearly inappropriate in some way to what is going on in the present.

Signs and symptoms of transference

◆ The client becomes inexplicably touchy, angry or sad, when we can see little apparent cause, or reacts strongly to some small comment or event.

◆ The client attributes feelings or actions to the therapist which the therapist doesn't believe are theirs.

◆ The therapist feels manoeuvred into reacting in ways which don't feel characteristic or which they would not have chosen.

Suggested courses of action

◆ Take time to think through what happened, and how you felt and reacted. In particular, think about how the particular interaction began – what actions or comments led up to it. Are there any clues there? If you know anything about the client's past, or about important relationships in the present, examine whether this incident resembles what the client has told you, or you have deduced, about patterns in those relationships. Did you trigger something or push an old button?

◆ Discuss the incident respectfully with the client, remembering to use words like 'wonder' and 'perhaps' and 'maybe' to present a suggestion rather than a direct interpretation – after all, you don't know.

◆ Discuss the event in your next supervision or with an impartial colleague or friend.

If the incident was puzzling or in any way fraught, you would probably be wise to discuss it with a supervisor or colleague before raising it again with the client. Someone with more experience – or simply the extra distance – can help us to see things which our own involvement may hide or blind us to. Checking out possible meanings and discussing the merits of various ways to handle the situation can be really helpful.

Transference can occur in any therapy, and hands-on therapies often allow the client to feel sheltered, nurtured and taken care of in ways that are reminiscent of childhood, thus potentially enhancing a child–parent dimension in the client–therapist relationship.

Touch itself reminds the person of past touching. An extreme case which body therapists may encounter at some time in their practice is a sudden physical response of aversion or tensing, coupled perhaps with tears or an expression of anger or distaste. This is likely to take the therapist by surprise, and in some cases may also puzzle the client. Children who have been physically traumatised may develop a helpful amnesia, but therapeutic touch in adulthood can sometimes break through this 'forgetting' because the body itself has been reminded of awareness in a certain area – even though that awareness is gentle and helpful in intent. A wise trainer we know once said: 'Muscles have memories'. This kind of acute response is discussed in more detail in Chapter 8.

 A client arrives 10 minutes late for an appointment. You comment jokingly: 'Missed the bus again, Mrs Jones?' The client bursts into tears. How do you respond?

You have been seeing a client for a number of months and their condition is now improving. Having spaced out the last few appointments to check that progress is continuing with less frequent intervention, you close a session by suggesting that the client may not need any further appointments. The client's face falls and they mutter in response: 'Well, I suppose if you have more urgent cases to treat…' What do you think might be causing this response and how do you deal with it?

A client tells you at the first consultation that they have seen a number of other practitioners, each of whom has failed to help them. You become aware after a number of sessions that your suggestions for homework and your encouraging comments on progress are being met with reasons why the client can't do as asked, or why the 'improvement' is not likely to last. You begin to feel impatient with the client, and are wondering if their view of the situation might not be correct after all. What might be happening here?

Counter-transference

Of course, the process of bringing the past into the present doesn't only happen to clients. It is a general feature of human behaviour. In everyday life we are often not aware of it, except when things go wrong and we get crossed wires or unexpected reactions. As therapists, however, we need to be aware of transference and our own version of exactly the same thing, because of the use or damage it can cause to the therapy. Psychotherapists may encourage the client's intensity of involvement, believing that it is a powerful medium for re-experiencing and then changing old and dysfunctional patterns. Body workers obviously have a different kind of training, but can nonetheless use the interaction surrounding their primary therapy with greater, or lesser, degrees of sensitivity and skill.

Where the therapist inadvertently imports their own material into the therapy, it may have confusing or potentially limiting effects. As always, self-monitoring and regular discussion with helpful outsiders is an important counterbalance.

Signs and symptoms of counter-transference

Counter-transference is indicated in cases where:

◆ the therapist is aware of difficulty in maintaining a professional stance towards the client (anger, impatience, overconcern and envy may all be indicators of a loss of objective distance)

◆ some event in the therapy precipitates an unexpected reaction in the therapist

◆ the therapist finds themself reluctant to discuss an issue or to consider something with a particular client, or with many clients, even though the therapy would seem to indicate it

◆ certain events regularly cause anxiety or distress in the therapist.

A single common denominator of all these is *the extent and degree of emotion felt by the therapist,* since any strong emotion tells us we have somehow shifted from our professional role into something more personal. While our personal feelings, of course, inform and enrich our professional life, it is when they seem to predominate that we should become alert to the possibility that our professional helpfulness may be being compromised. *It is important to recognise that strength of 'good' or positive feelings may be just as compromising of the professional relationship as more negative feelings.*

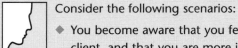

Consider the following scenarios:

◆ You become aware that you feel very sorry for a particular client, and that you are more indulgent towards them in boundary matters, e.g. lateness and late cancellations, than you are towards other clients.

◆ You find that you are looking forward to a particular client's visits.

◆ A client tells you that since their last session their mother has become seriously ill. You spend some time discussing and sympathising with their anxiety, telling the client how you managed to cope with a similar situation some years ago. You feel very flat during the rest of the day, and guilty that you have not been your usual cheery self with other clients.

> ◆ You notice that whenever a client cancels an appointment you feel quite anxious about whether you will get enough work that week. Your receptionist comments that you were quite brusque to one client phoning in to cancel – 'What's bitten her today?' you hear her saying to another colleague as you return to your room.
>
> Take time to consider in each case what the therapist might be projecting into the situation and how they could deal with it.
>
> 1. What might they need to do for themself (see also Chs 15 and 16)?
>
> 2. How best might they deal with the client?

Sexual issues

A working relationship between therapist and client is most effective where it is focused on their shared therapeutic goal, however nurturing the context. But, as we have said, because the relationship is between two unique people – and this is the basis of its value to both – issues of sexuality and sexual attraction do from time to time colour the relationship, even if they do not become explicit. This may involve people of the same gender as well as opposite genders.

We want to look at some common fears experienced by each party, and then at issues arising where a mutual attraction is felt. In reflecting on actions and feelings in the therapy, it is important for the therapist to monitor what is implied as well as overt, drawing upon the wealth of social 'instinct' which we have already emphasised as being one of our most useful resources.

Common fears of the therapist

Some common fears are:

◆ that the client will constantly bring conversation towards a sexual base or innuendo

◆ that the client will explicitly indicate that sexual favours are being sought or would be welcomed

◆ that an actual sexual advance/attack will be made.

In our experience, both the fears and the actual instances can occur to therapists of either sex and in both heterosexual and homosexual interactions.

Monitoring what is going on at a variety of levels in the interaction allows the therapist to begin to become alert to possible patterns. With experience, this becomes more automatic, but in early days of practice it is worth training oneself to reflect at the end of a session on verbal or behavioural cues the client may be offering. If you find you have felt uncomfortable with a particular client, ask what cues have led to this feeling. Have you perhaps 'ignored' a number of innuendos or sexually flavoured jokes? Has the client come into your personal space 'accidentally'? Ignoring such signals does not make them go away and it may allow a client to believe, or convince themself, that their behaviour is acceptable. You might find it useful to rehearse a number of possible responses, both verbal and non-verbal, which could indicate that you are not prepared to accept a sexual overtone to the therapy. Again, you could discuss the events and your perception of them in supervision or with a trusted outsider, to check whether you are being oversensitive or fearful.

Addressing implicit signals may allow you to re-establish the therapeutic base more neutrally. It is also likely to prevent overt advances from being made, since most people will test the reaction before proceeding further. If you don't react when someone tells a questionable joke or 'accidentally' touches your bottom as they pass you, they may well take this as being an invitation to more explicit advances.

A good example might be a patient attempting to chat up a young female doctor, getting very close to her and asking why she doesn't seem to want them to be friends. She could reply, without any hostility, 'I've got plenty of friends, thank you', while firmly moving away.

The worst fear a therapist may have is of a client making a sexual advance or attack. If you have trusted your ability to evaluate the client from the outset (see Ch. 3), this is very unlikely, as you will already have rejected some possible clients because you felt some discomfort or unease about them. Even if you decided to take the client on, you may have alerted your receptionist to your doubts about them or, if working at home, arranged for someone else to be in the house during their session.

We do not want to imply that attack is likely; but in the same way as we sensibly take out insurance against various risks, we should try to ensure that the circumstances of our practice and our behaviour minimise risk, and monitor behaviour and reactions in the personal aspects of our interaction with the client with just as much care as we monitor their response to our treatment.

One specific event which female bodyworkers often fear is a male client developing an erection. *The problem is not the erection, but what led up to it.* If there has been no previous indication of mental or physical sexual interest from the client towards the therapist, the situation can be ignored. Bodies respond to touch with differing degrees of sensitivity, and a number of clients – of both sexes – have told us how embarrassed they felt on becoming aroused in the presence of a therapist, even where the therapist did not see their reaction. It is important, if the client does know you have seen them, that you treat the event matter-of-factly and without blame or embarrassment – it is their problem. You might ask if they would like you to leave the room for a short while or if they would like to turn over.

If there has been any verbal or physical indication of sexual interest before, and you have dealt with it professionally, you need to indicate your concern and point out that their interest is inappropriate in the context of therapy. You may need at this point to suggest that therapy with you should be discontinued since its effectiveness has been seriously compromised.

Physical arousal in a female client may be less noticeable, although engorgement of erectile tissue such as the nipples could be an indicator if the client is undressed. Clearly, the response is inappropriate to a therapeutic context, but the client does not need chastising or blaming. We need to remember that the very inappropriateness of the response indicates a need or problem in the client, for which they may need a different kind of help.

Both blaming and accepting the response compound the problem.

Common fears of clients

Some common fears are:

◆ exposing private parts of the body

◆ inappropriate touching

◆ verbal sexual advances

◆ physical sexual advances

◆ breaking wind.

There are many reasons for clients to have these fears. These range from learned inhibitions common to many, or most, people from their upbringing to specific anxieties resulting from abuse. It is important in our behaviour with all clients to base our behaviour on the safest, least intrusive level – to treat all clients initially with the sensitivity appropriate to someone who does have reason to be fearful. This leads us to provide privacy for clients to dress and undress (being absent from the room while they do it, or having special cubicles or screens), keeping a clear physical distance from them if not actually working hands-on, and conveying a professional neutrality in the very way we do our hands-on work.

Another important dimension of our interaction which needs to be reassuringly non-sexual is our language. We need to avoid double meanings and to be aware that humour, too, can give unwanted messages. As we build up rapport with individual clients, we learn more about their safety margins, and with many we can become more spontaneous and less rigid in our neutrality than we needed to be at the outset. But being aware that it is our responsibility to define the relationship and make it a safe context for the client needs to be a primary concern throughout treatment.

Sexual attraction

So far, we have looked at unwanted, unreciprocated, sexual response in therapy. More insidious in some ways is attraction felt by either or both, since it seems less threatening.

Therapist attracted to client

Such an attraction will inevitably compromise therapy because you will have lost your professional distance, however much you try to kid yourself that it doesn't! We believe the only honest course you can take here is to refer the client to another therapist. You will need to give the client a reason for the referral.

Acceptable reasons are:

◆ that you have reached the limits of your skill in helping them

◆ that somebody else has even more skills to meet their need

◆ the truth (though this will depend on the strength of your professional relationship with the client). Referring them on allows you both to consider what you want to do next as private individuals.

Client attracted to therapist

If your client is attracted to you:

◆ Be prepared to acknowledge it to yourself. What makes you think that this is the case (evidence, verbal and non-verbal)?

◆ Check the evidence. Reflect on other possible examples. Ask yourself whether the behaviour you have identified might equally indicate dependency in the client.

◆ Discuss the case in supervision/with a colleague or trusted outsider.

◆ Discuss the possibility with the client, while making it clear that no blame is attached: 'It sometimes happens that clients feel attracted to their therapists. I'm beginning to wonder if you might be feeling something like that...'

◆ If you feel uncomfortable, or if the client does as a result of the discussion, consider terminating therapy. Make it clear that the reason for ending therapy is that attraction complicates and compromises the effectiveness of the therapy itself. Reassure the client that this is not a rejection of them as a person (but at the same time, don't give them grounds to hope for a personal involvement after the therapy ends unless you genuinely want one). Be aware that a client's feelings of attraction to the therapist may be very genuine at the time, but can often be provoked by the combination of dependence, vulnerability and special attention in the situation itself.

Mutual attraction

In this case:

◆ consider the evidence and acknowledge what is happening

◆ discuss in supervision

◆ decide where you would like the relationship to go

◆ discuss with the client, but not during actual treatment.

Even if the client does not wish to continue the relationship on a personal basis, despite the attraction, you should probably terminate the therapy for all the reasons already discussed, as its effectiveness will have been compromised.

In all the situations we have discussed in this chapter, our prime concern as therapists is to maintain the integrity of the therapeutic context we offer our clients. This means training ourselves to monitor honestly our ability to remain caring, concerned and involved with our clients, but within a firmly professional role which maintains safety and trust. Their business in being with us is to benefit from our professional skill, mediated through our individual personality and approach. Anything which compromises this careful context threatens the success of our work together.

13 ⬥ Record-keeping and confidential filing

The final part of the therapist–client interaction is the taking and storing of notes. The keeping of records is a vital element of the treatment process, charting the client's progress and informing future treatment. It also acts as insurance should a client take issue with a particular aspect of treatment, allege an unpleasant reaction as a result of treatment or complain that a therapist acted improperly.

Most complementary therapy associations issue notes of guidance concerning note-taking and the storage of records and these should be followed. This chapter is not meant to replace advice given during training or supersede notes of guidance, but rather to act as a complement.

Record-keeping is a process, and the first part of the process is about deciding when to take notes. The other parts cover the type of information to be recorded (and who, if anybody, has access), where records are to be kept and for how long.

When to record

It is likely that you will start taking notes from your first telephone contact, i.e. name, address, telephone number, presenting concerns, possible symptoms, etc. These pieces of information will form the basis of the case history that you will take during your first consultation.

During the initial consultation you will be requesting detailed information which you will be recording as it is delivered. You will therefore need to be clear in your questioning, provide the client with time and space to think, and be able to hear their replies.

A useful technique is to ask the question, observe and listen to the client's reply, feed back what you believe you have heard and then record it. This guarantees that you record the correct information, without any interpretation or mishearing. It also provides the client with the opportunity to check that they are comfortable with what has been said and add to it or clarify it should they feel it necessary.

This part of the note-taking process is straightforward; the client will be expecting you to take a case history (from your initial telephone contact and/or your literature) and therefore to take notes. How you carry this out initially could well set the scene for future note-taking. If it is carried out sensitively and unobtrusively and the client does not feel interrupted or disregarded, then they will see your taking notes as a positive experience (see Ch. 5 for ideas on seating, type of information needed, questioning etc.).

During subsequent treatments, you will need to decide when to undertake note-taking. Do you make notes during the first 10 minutes – noting how the client has been since the last treatment, recurring patterns of behaviour, symptoms, etc. – or after the treatment is completed, or both? If you wish to take notes during the first 10 minutes, do explain your reasons to your client and check that they are accepted: 'I would like to take notes as we go along but if you feel that this would be intrusive then please say so.'

Some clients do not like notes being taken when they are talking. They feel that the therapist's attention is more focused on taking down the information than listening to what is continuing to be said. So do check. It may be helpful to the client to explain that taking notes at the time means that all the relevant information is recorded whilst it is fresh.

Obviously the decision about when to take notes rests on the degree and nature of the information to be recorded, how comfortable or otherwise your client feels about the process, and your own preferences; these may well differ from one client to another.

The 'when' of note-taking could also be influenced by the therapist's own state of well-being. If you have had a tiring day and feel that your concentration is in danger of slipping, or that your ability to retain information is not at its best, then it may well be that you decide to seek your client's permission to take notes from the outset: 'Would you mind if I took notes as we went along today? I am concerned to make an accurate record of what has been happening since we last met.'

You may well have experimented with note-taking when you were carrying out your case studies, in which case you may already have preferences and information as to what works for you and what doesn't. What is important is that you stay flexible in your approach in order that the client is not left feeling that note-taking has interrupted their train of thought or flow of speech.

The final part of note-taking takes place after treatment, when you record what treatment was carried out, what you noted, difficulties experienced possibly due to body condition or client concerns, etc. If you did not take notes during the first 10 minutes of the session then any pertinent information will need to be recorded at this juncture. Your notes can be started when the client is dressing, and subsequently completed when they have left, but, as far as possible, before the next client arrives. If this does not suit your style of therapy and mode of treatment delivery then good practice decrees that your records are completed as soon as possible after the client has left your treatment room. The longer you leave your recording, the more likely you are to forget important pieces of information or to muddle what happened in one client's treatment with another! Records should be completed the same day.

Type of information to record

You will need to record information that is pertinent to the client's condition and treatment. It will be important to base your recording on evidence rather than opinion. (This is not to say that the therapist should not voice opinions, but they need to be based on specifics that can be substantiated, not on assumptions and prejudice.)

As well as charting the change or otherwise of presenting symptoms, it will be important to note if there are patterns of behaviour or attitudes, or lifestyle changes/fluctuations that influence the client's progress. (You will need to look at how you help the client to explore these issues and use their new knowledge positively to influence their situation.)

What do you do if a client tells you that they are taking illegal drugs (or are involved in any other illegal activity)? Do you record the information? We feel that it will be important to do so if you or your client feel that it is contributing – positively or negatively – to their condition. If it is not an influencing factor, a discussion with your client as to the purpose of giving you the information will be important. What were they expecting you to do? What will you do? It could be that they hoped that you and your therapy would be able to support them in changing their behaviours, or that you might refuse to treat them, thereby acting as a motivator for change. Our suggestion is that you discuss it with the client and then your supervisor. If you do not have a supervisor then consult another professional or your professional association. If all that fails, seek guidance from the British Medical Association (BMA) or the British Association of Counselling (BAC).

In certain circumstances, you may need to inform other agencies, such as GP practice, social services or the police. This would most certainly apply to any information that denoted that harm or injury was being inflicted on, or likely to occur to, another person. You will need to inform your client about your actions before you pass on the information, and also make it clear why you are passing on information.

In all of the above, it will be important that you follow your association's guidelines, take advice and record thoroughly.

Who has access to client information?

Other than in the scenarios highlighted above, the client needs to give permission for a therapist to discuss confidential information with a third party. When taking a case history, it is common practice to take the name and address of the GP and, depending upon the condition being treated, to seek permission to make contact should it be felt advisable. In such circumstances, only the information relevant to the medical condition should be discussed.

It is now common practice for everyone to have access to their medical records and the therapist should be prepared to adopt the same policy. This means that the information should be clearly recorded and, as stated earlier in the chapter, based on evidence or opinion that can be substantiated.

It is good practice to explain to clients at the outset whether you have a supervisor and what it means. Let them know that it is a routine and helpful part of supervision to discuss cases, i.e. that it is a confidential exchange with another professional which ultimately benefits the therapist and the client.

Storage

In its code of practice, the BAC states that all written notes should be kept under lock and key, and most other professional associations also make this stipulation. The reason is self-evident. A filing cabinet or other lockable container should be used, with the key stored in a safe, non-public place. The normal time for records to be kept is a minimum of 5 years. After this period, you may dispose of them, but they must be shredded or burned to ensure lasting confidentiality.

The Data Protection Act

If you decide to keep full records on a computer, please be mindful of the Data Protection Act and whether you need to register. Every data user who holds personal data that is processed by a computer must be registered unless all the data falls within certain exemptions. It is most likely that you, as a therapist, will be required to register. The cost to register is currently £75.00.

The Act (1984) was introduced because of concerns about individuals' rights of personal privacy in the light of the then rapidly developing computer technology. The Act is administered by the Office of the Data Protection Registrar and is concerned with 'personal data which is automatically processed'. The Act for the first time set out the rights that an individual has concerning information stored about them on a computer; it also sets out the responsibilities of the users of the data.

There are eight data protection principles. Data must be:

1. obtained and processed fairly and lawfully

2. held only for the lawful purposes described in the register entry

3. used only for those purposes and only be disclosed to those people described in the register entry

4. adequate, relevant and not excessive in relation to the purpose for which it is held

5. accurate and where necessary kept up to date (content)

6. held no longer than is necessary for the registered purpose (time element)

7. accessible to the individual concerned who has the right to have information about themselves corrected or erased (access issue)

8. surrounded by proper security.

If the data user fails to follow these principles then the registrar may take action against the data user.

Information on the DPA can be obtained through a free booklet called the *Data Protection Guidelines* and can be ordered by telephoning the registrar's enquiry service on 01625 545745 or by faxing on 01625 524510.

Record-keeping is an essential part of your therapy, not an additional chore. As part of your work with an individual, it requires the same efficiency and sensitivity as you observe in the rest of your practice. Done properly it benefits both you and your client.

14 ► Time-keeping and payment

Since our theme throughout the book is that the working structure within which therapy takes place also conveys messages, it follows that time-keeping and payment are a potent source of information. They have an essential and guiding place in establishing the rules of engagement in the therapy for both parties, which allows them to demonstrate a mutual respect and sense of dignity, each with their own contribution.

In arriving at decisions about cost, time frame and what might need to be done to encourage the client to keep to agreed procedures, the therapist is in fact debating issues of self-worth. In their response to the boundaries within which the therapy takes place, the client is offering enacted information about themselves, their helper and the likelihood of therapeutic change.

All this may seem very heavy, and newly qualified therapists can find these apparently mercenary or organisational issues difficult or distasteful to consider. We want in this chapter to offer some help in understanding why these factors are important, and some very practical, rule-of-thumb suggestions for managing them effectively.

The reluctant therapist

Setting rules can put the therapist in mind of parental and instructional roles: telling people how much they have to pay and what will happen if they come late or make a late cancellation can feel very different from the caring, gentle approach they see as being 'really' therapeutic. It may feel easier to let something go by without commenting than to take issue with the client about it.

It may be useful here to think about helpful parents and teachers you may have known. We believe that helpfulness involves clarity and firmness about rules as well as caring and support.

> Think about some rule-setting you have experienced. Find some examples that you found helpful, where the rule-setter helped you to understand the necessity – or advantages – of keeping to the rule. How did they do it? Think about the words, the tone of voice, and whether they explained what might happen if the rule was kept/not kept? Now think of some examples which left you unclear, where a rule suddenly appeared after you had already broken it, or where the explanation made you angry or resentful. Try to identify what characterised these interactions. How did the two differ from each other?

We have all been on the receiving end of both good and bad rule-setting and boundary-keeping. One client described the effect of poor boundary-keeping by her parents as being 'like walking on glass' – she never knew when she would be injured or how severely.

As a therapist, we share something with parents and teachers: it is our job to create a clear and caring context within which the client can be helped to recover or to change and grow. Being clear about boundaries actually simplifies the task of helping, because it means we can put our major energies into the therapeutic work rather than into uncertainties or debates about contractual or structural detail. (Developing a habit of homework/washing up or some other household task allows energy to be conserved or directed profitably into the task rather than into arguments about the doing of it.)

One of the reasons why we often find it difficult to set prices and rules to start with is that when we are only recently qualified we feel unsure of our ability and certainly unfamiliar with our new-found status as 'expert'. We are still emotionally within the student mode, with all its awareness of more to understand, of skills as yet unlearnt and of experience not had.

One very wise tutor we knew regularly used to remind students in training that even though they had not yet qualified, they could already be confident that they could offer something valuable to their clients – their time and their undivided attention. Most people only very rarely have the experience of someone else's undivided attention for an hour, let alone a longer period. The development of a body of expertise over and above this makes even the newest therapist valuable to a client in need.

If your course involved some help with setting up a practice, you will already have considered how to set a fee for your work. If you are working in a clinic, the clinic will have benchmarked fees according to local norms. Be sure in yourself that you are worth every penny. You can put your fees up towards the top of the local range as you get more experience, but even at the outset you need to get into the habit of seeing yourself as deserving at least as much as the norm for your therapy in your area. If you have been a client yourself, and know how helpful you have found the help you were given, you may find it easier to imagine how your clients will value you. Remember, too, that in choosing to ask for help and in choosing you as their therapist, they are choosing to opt in to their part of the contract. You don't need to persuade them – only yourself! (If you do need to persuade them, it may be worth consulting Ch. 6 on involving the client in the process.)

One of the most normal things about people is that we can imagine vividly the things we fear. If we feel unconfident, we anticipate the very difficulties we would most like to avoid. So we are inclined to be apologetic about contract and boundary setting, and especially about boundary enforcement. We shudder at the very thought of what to say to a client who has a session and then realises that they have left their cash and cheque book behind. It can seem easier in the circumstances to say 'Oh, don't worry' than to ask them simply and firmly to deliver the payment later that evening, or to put in the post next morning. But what happens next time? Do you remind them that they now owe you for two sessions? Do you wait for them to remember? What if both of you forget? What if you duck out of reminding them and they only offer for one? It can be a minefield quite unnecessarily entered into. Clients find it confusing too. And the uncertainty and unease then gets in the way of the therapeutic exchange between you.

Like most people who have been in practice for some time, we have each had our share of uncomfortable experiences around money and boundary issues, and a few bad debts (see later in the chapter for ways to minimise these). It is partly from our own uncomfortable moments that we have become very sure that simple and clear rule-setting and firm boundary maintenance help both therapist and client to know where they are and to get on with the real business of the therapy.

The value to the client

The client benefits from clear rules and boundaries in another way, too. Clients often seek help when they are in need of more than just physical treatment. Sometimes illness or accident are part of ongoing life crises – caused by stress, perhaps, or by the body enacting the conflicts or uncertainties in their emotional life. Sometimes chronic physical problems are the cause of relationship problems or depression. In asking for help to relax or to treat a physical problem, the client is putting themself in a context where they feel supported and, by unconscious implication, able to change. The treatment situation is a microcosm of their life – they bring their feelings, their fears, their attitudes and their behaviours as well as their rigid back or unlevel pelvis, their IBS or frequent migraines. Giving them the experience of clear boundaries and uncomplicated interaction is a way of implying that life can be clearer and less complicated. Involving them in making and maintaining a clean, functioning contract to work together, and working straightforwardly and honestly through any problems that may arise, is one way of demonstrating through experience that they can be a partner in a healthy interaction.

Self-audit

As a useful next step, ask yourself which contractual areas you have reluctance about, or have previously experienced difficulties in. We have identified some common ones, and will go on to look at some ways of managing each effectively:

◆ setting a fee

◆ putting up fees

◆ deciding whether or not to reduce or waive costs

◆ payment by third parties

◆ bad debts

◆ last-minute cancellations

◆ clients who argue or quibble

◆ clients who arrive late

◆ overrunning time yourself

◆ clients who are 'high maintenance'

◆ dealing with your own mistakes in administration or treatment.

Setting a fee

Your fee should relate to:

◆ the norm for your area

◆ the length of session

- ◆ the nature of the treatment (e.g. whole body massage vs. neck and shoulder)

- ◆ whether the session is an initial one or a continuation (may affect length; also first session can be more demanding for the therapist)

- ◆ how experienced/highly qualified you are

- ◆ any reductions you have decided to make, e.g. for block booking, for an unemployed client or a child.

Start by finding out the norm for a typical length session for your type of therapy in your area and work from there. You have to feel able to ask confidently for your fee – but, equally, it is no good feeling that you have undersold yourself.

Putting up fees

As you acquire more experience or further qualifications, and as time goes by and the cost of living rises, you will need to put your fee up. This need may already confront you if you have been charging a small fee as a student in training and now need to begin charging the full rate to people who have been your practice clients. In this case, you may actually have a harder job than you will have at later stages in your career, since the jump from a student fee (perhaps expenses only) to a full professional charge is larger than most later increases. This means that future increases will be a lot easier!

Again, the first person to convince is yourself. In acquiring a full qualification, and later, more experience, you are worth more to the client. Your knowledge base is greater; your skills more fluent and adept. Remind yourself of the differences between now and when you began, now and the early days of your training (now and when you first qualified). You will have raised your own expectations and ambitions, of course, but look back for a moment. How much extra are you worth?

Find a convenient amount. Bear in mind that people bringing cash will have to find notes or coins, and that for a day's full work you may have to supply yourself with a stack of change. For this reason, put your fee up in 50p or £1 amounts, and every so often be realistic and put it up by a larger amount, e.g. £5.

Give sufficient warning. If you are nearing the end of your training, tell your practice clients when you will be qualifying and what you will be charging after qualification. You could let them know how this relates to the norm for your area. You can put your fee up in stages, if you think it will be easier for them to get used to. Because this jump is the largest you are likely to have to make, you will need to give longer warning than when you are raising a fully professional fee by a few pounds (most people will accept a jump of up to £5 if they have experienced and value your work). Once in practice, you can either warn all clients that your fee will go up from a set date (put up a notice in your consulting room, send out a card) or you can tell each one as they come that your fee will be increased from their next session (or the one after). This second option is a little messier to manage and you will need to jot down the revised fee against their name in your book when you make the next appointment; but the advantage is that you can roll the rise and more easily make exceptions. For example, if a client is nearing the end of their work with you, you may decide to let them finish at the old rate, or if you feel they are already stretching their purse to find the old rate, you can leave the fee as it is. It's harder to do this if you have a public notice in the waiting room. On the other hand, putting the fee up all at once is a lot simpler. It is your practice and your choice.

Once you have decided to put your fee up, be clear and don't apologise or offer too much in the way of explanation or justification. Remember Shakespeare's comment in Hamlet: 'Methinks the lady doth protest too much'. Give a brief reason, if there is one the client will understand:

> *'Since I'll be qualified after Easter...'*

> *'The cost of oils has been going up over the last few years and I have to put my fee up now to cover those increases...'*

> *'I've held my fee for the last 2 years, but now I need to increase it in line with the cost of living rises...'*

Deciding whether or not to reduce or waive costs

Having set your normal fee, you need a policy about exceptions. If you are working in a clinic, the clinic probably has its own policy and you can borrow this for your private practice if you think it useful. If you are self-employed, working from your own or clients' homes, it is up to you. You need to take into consideration:

◆ the kinds of clients you anticipate working with

◆ their ability to pay your normal rate

◆ the commitment implied in paying (see Ch. 3)

◆ having a system which is simple for you to run.

If you think that some of the people you want to work with may not be able to afford your full fee (e.g. because they are unemployed or on a low income), you can have a special rate for these categories. When people enquire about your fee, you can give them both rates. This makes it easier for them – it is not easy to plead poverty and leaving it to the client to ask if you do a reduced rate may put some off.

It is important, though, that they pay something. If you are self-employed, you may from time to time wish to take a client for a notional payment only because you feel they need your help even though they cannot afford it. As we said before, even a token payment represents a commitment and maintains the client's self-esteem and dignity.

On a more mundane level, it is probably simpler to have a tariff with only two levels, rather than a more complicated one, knowing that you can also make individual, one-off exceptions. As you get busier, administrative simplicity gets more important for your diary and your accounts. For example, imagine the hassle of putting up your fees if you have different clients paying a number of different rates. Do you put everyone up a couple of pounds? Do you round everyone up to the nearest even number?

Payment by third parties

We suggest that you consider third-party payment as a norm for children, and only accept it in exceptional cases for anyone else. The contract becomes messy with someone else involved and it can lead to a lack of clarity about who you are accountable to. For example, both you and the client may find yourselves feeling the need to justify continued treatment (perhaps on a winding-down or maintenance basis) if someone else is paying, whereas if the client were responsible for their own payment, they could make that decision about need versus finance themselves. Obviously, some people will only be able to come if effectively financed by someone else. Non-working women are a good example of this, and they often feel beholden to their bread-winning partner and may curtail therapy as soon as there is a significant improvement rather than continuing as long as they, and you, feel is really ideal.

For this reason, when you see the client for the first time, try to find out tactfully if they feel under any pressure about where the money is coming from. For your part, be as clear as you can about how long the therapy might last and what the costs are likely to be – you would do this anyway, but you can talk explicitly with the client about the importance of their 'owning' the therapy and not being unduly pressured by people in the wings.

Sometimes a friend or family member other than a partner offers to pay. If your therapy is a relaxing one (e.g. massage), this may come as a treat – the payer may make the arrangement beforehand with you or they may give the client the money to give you. These gifts rarely cause the kind of difficulties we are taking about. Where someone wishes to enter into medium- or long-term therapy to treat a medical condition but needs someone else to finance it, we suggest you explain the reasons why it is important that the contract effectively remains between them and you. The simplest way of managing this is for the client to pay you directly, by cash or cheque, and for their sponsor to provide them with the money in whatever way they agree – a cheque made out to you, cash or reimbursement of the client afterwards. You can help the client to find a clear and simple means to explain why this is a good way to arrange things, as it is quite likely that they and their sponsor may not have thought about it.

This is also a good practice in the case of teenagers, as it helps to maintain their dignity as your client and may create a constructive distance between the therapy and a possibly overinvolved or controlling parent. Do not argue the case with the parent, if it is the parent who talks with you at the outset. Simply tell them this is how you arrange things as you have found it clearer and simpler for all concerned.

Bad debts

The best way to deal with these is not to get any. Even the most experienced practitioners, however, have had a few in their time. We believe that the following simple rules will help to minimise their likelihood; but if you do find that someone at some time gets through the net *do not give yourself a bad time about it and do not hang onto the resentment.* That way, you would have lost out twice, whereas if you put it down to experience and try to learn from it, the client has only got away with your money, not your peace of mind. Hence:

◆ Ask for payment at the end of each session.

◆ If the client has 'forgotten' the money or cheque, ask them to deliver it by hand or put it in the post first class *the same day.* If the payment fails to arrive, phone the client as soon as you can to enquire/remind them.

◆ Make any further appointments conditional upon payment having been received first – if you have any doubts about the client's intention to pay (if it seems to be more than a simple forgetting), don't even put a further appointment in your book until you have been paid.

If the worst happens, you will only have lost payment for one session. In this case, make it clear to the client in writing that they have forfeited their right to treatment with you. In an exceptional case, you could resume treatment if you have reason to believe that the client will be reliable in future, but we suggest that in this case you ask for payment in advance.

If this seems hard, remember that condoning improper dealing *does not help the client.* If you ignore the behaviour, the unintended message to the client could be that you are condoning it. Unconscious or deliberate stealing of therapy may indicate deeper personal or interpersonal problems which need help (probably from some form of psychotherapy). If you expect, and as far as humanly possible ensure, mutually respectful interaction with your clients, you will be helping them in an important way quite apart from your overt therapy.

Last-minute cancellations

Cancellations happen – a client (or one of their relatives) gets ill; a meeting is rearranged; something has to be done in a hurry. All good reasons. You need a clear policy, which relates to the inconvenience caused to you and your practice.

If the cancellation is well ahead of time, inconvenience is minimal and you will be able to rearrange the appointment and fill the empty slot.

The nearer the time of the appointment, the less chance you have of giving the appointment to another client. This has two effects: first, even clients who are wanting an appointment may not be able to take advantage of the space because they can't rearrange their commitments to make the time available; and second, you may end up losing earnings even though with longer notice you could have filled the space. In this case, it is quite reasonable to ask for a cancellation fee. You will need to warn clients at the outset that this could happen. Most people understand the situation, particularly when you remind them that other clients wanting treatment are as much inconvenienced as you are, but no-one wants to be told at the last moment that there is a penalty to be paid. You can either warn them when making the very first appointment – 'Oh, and you need to know that if you ever need to cancel at the last moment, I may have to ask you to pay for the session' – or you can incorporate a brief written explanation into your business leaflet or next-appointment card. You might do both. If you are able to fill the space at the last moment, it is clearly not ethical to charge the cancellation fee. If the client cancels because of illness or accident, you may want to interpret your rule generously. You are probably glad not to see them if they have flu or a heavy cold, so it may be better to lose the fee than earn it with some attendant germs. If they have crashed their car, or a relative has taken an overdose, their life is hard enough without extra penalties. *If in doubt, imagine how you would feel in their situation and ask what you would think fair treatment from your therapist.*

If a cancellation fee is appropriate, you can ask all or part of the full fee. Depending on the situation and the client, you may tell them they can add the cancellation fee to the payment for their next session, or alternatively ask them to send it to you sooner (paying for two sessions at once can make a hole in the budget and feel like a lot even if the client agrees it is fair).

Clients who argue or quibble

Most of us dislike conflict. As we said in Chapter 3, you get lots of important information even in initial enquiries, and you may begin to feel even then that a client is likely to be 'difficult'. Try to work out what the difficulty is about. Are they aggressive in questioning the effectiveness of your therapy or your qualifications? Are they quibbling about the expense? Do they leap in right away and ask if you ever do deals for multiple sessions or 'joke' about cost in some way? Even if you answer their questions clearly and confidently, and they do not pursue the issue, this may be an indicator of problems to come. *Don't let yourself be persuaded into any arrangement or modification of your normal rules unless you really feel it is acceptable; and don't let yourself be bullied. It is not worth taking on a bullying client.* You may allow the discussion to go on a little longer just to check that your impression is borne out by the client's continued behaviour. If it is, find the politest way you can to avoid taking them on.

You may well feel upset, angry or resentful about this afterwards. Give yourself some time and space to think it through, and remind yourself that you only have a short-term bad feeling – the client may have a long-term problem.

Clients who arrive late

Most of us are late for an appointment from time to time. There are lots of reasons and most of them are quite understandable and therefore acceptable.

However, there are two kinds of lateness which are more problematic for the therapist: lateness which effectively curtails the available working time of the session and lateness which is habitual.

Occasionally a client may arrive late enough to effectively reduce the working length of the session. If this does not seem to be their fault, work out what you can do for them in the time that is left and discuss it with them so that you re-agree the contract for that day (e.g. a neck and shoulder massage rather than full body). It is still legitimate to charge them for the full time, since it was set aside for them and could not be used for anyone or anything else. If there is not enough time for physical treatment, take the opportunity to have a review discussion – how much progress has been made; where do you feel treatment needs to go next; how are the improvements showing up in the client's wider life? Review sessions have their place in ongoing treatment anyway, and even though this one may have been unscheduled, you can turn a potential disappointment into something useful to you both.

Where the client is regularly late, even by as little as 5–15 minutes, it may be useful to point it out to them and to ask them why they think this happens. If the difficulty seems structural – getting kids to school, waiting for a certain bus – it might be better to agree a different time for your sessions, rather than worrying about lateness or getting irritated by it. If the problem isn't functional in this way, it's worth asking the client if they are often, or usually, a little late for things in life. Sometimes lateness indicates a mild rebellion or lack of respect for the commitment, sometimes quite the opposite – a feeling of unworthiness for help or treatment. Discussing these possibilities in an open rather than an irritated way with the client and allowing them to realise that this pattern is quite common often brings to the surface important issues. Sometimes just having the discussion is enough to make the pattern change for the better, as the client can then address the underlying issue internally or in discussion with you or with family or other appropriate helpers. If there is a clear and repeated pattern don't ignore it, as this not only leaves the pattern untouched but makes you a partner in suffering from it! It may also have a knock-on effect on clients you see later in the day.

Overrunning time yourself

It takes time to acquire an accurate internal timer for your therapy. When you started to practise, it probably took you much longer to give a complete treatment than it does now, but you may still feel anxious about finishing the hands-on work, winding up the session and preparing yourself and your treatment room for the next client in time. Having an easily visible clock in the room, which you can glance at from time to time without being obtrusive about it, can help you pace your work in relation to the time available, and with practice you will get to know exactly what your finishing and turnaround time needs to be. Even so, there will be some occasions when you don't quite make it, and when your next client has to wait. You need to apologise to the client kept waiting and, if possible, offer to extend their session length by an appropriate amount. What if you have still another client after them? You don't want to keep them waiting too. You can:

◆ phone the third client and ask them if they can come a little later than arranged

◆ tell the second client that you unfortunately have to keep to time but offer a small reduction in the fee to compensate for the inconvenience; you may also need to explain briefly why you were late if the reasons were beyond your control (you had to deal with something unexpected in the treatment, or the client became upset)

◆ think about whether you need to build in a short non-accountable time (10 or 15 minutes, perhaps) between clients to prevent these problems occurring

◆ work out whether your treatment routine may need shortening or your session lengthening – the latter may not be possible if you work in a clinic.

Clients who are 'high maintenance'

Some clients demand more than others. They may change appointments frequently, leave phone messages with urgent questions and updates on progress ('I thought I ought to tell you...'), or give you important information just as they are about to leave ('By the way...'). While none of these behaviours in themselves necessarily indicates self-absorption, dependence or underlying psychological difficulties, they may. If a client's repeated behaviour involves more than one of these patterns, you are likely to begin to feel irritated, perhaps without quite knowing why, since each incident is often explainable or apparently justifiable. Taken together, however, you are experiencing a mild form of stress because the client is *pushing the boundaries of the therapy.*

You might deal with a high maintenance client as follows:

◆ Consider how the client strikes you overall. Do they seem anxious for reassurance? Have they adequate support networks apart from the therapy? Do they understand the process and aims of what you are doing with them? These things might indicate that the client is used to depending on others (perhaps specifically on people in authority roles) and is inviting you to offer more obvious or sustained support. It might be that you have underestimated their insecurity: ask yourself (perhaps also ask a colleague or supervisor) if it would help the client to 'firm up' your holding or supporting role a little.

◆ On the other hand, you might also consider whether the client is now needing to become more independent and self-reliant. If you feel this is the case, try to work out how to combine a continuing warmth and reassurance that they can cope with some targets or tasks for which they can be responsible and which they can report back on at your next session. You could explain to the client that you feel this will help them to begin to take more control of their own progress.

◆ If you feel that the client is demanding your time and attention for psychological reasons, this may indicate that they have a difficulty or pattern which needs explicit psychological help. In any event, it will not help them to allow unreasonable demands (e.g. phoning you incessantly at home or leaving lots of messages with a clinic receptionist which require your reply). When you next see the client, make it clear that this level of demand is going beyond what an individual client has a right to expect, but that you understand that the questions and contact are important to them. You could remind them that your expertise is in the treatment of physical conditions and suggest that counselling or psychological help might help them.

Dealing with your own mistakes in administration or treatment

Administration

At some time in their careers, virtually all therapists will make some kind of administrative mistake: forgetting or double-booking an appointment; losing a client's notes; forgetting to inform a client of changed arrangements; not phoning back in response to a telephone message. All these are typical errors which can inconvenience the client and potentially make them feel irritated, disappointed and let down. However good your reasons, apologise as sincerely as you are able, and try to correct or make amends for the error. Being human, the client will also have made this kind of error at some time themselves, and straightforward confession and apology will go far towards restoring a good relationship between you.

Errors in treatment

Hopefully, your training and good practice, and the support systems you have around you (see Ch. 16) will make this kind of error unlikely. However, if you feel you have made a mistake, or if a client believes you have, you need to remain as calm and professional as you can.

Sometimes a disappointed or angry client will make even the most level-tempered therapist feel defensive when an error is pointed out. The sillier we feel, the easier it is to respond defensively. We know of one therapist who, through inexperience with a particular procedure, used it unskilfully and caused the client considerable distress. The client found herself becoming angrier in the interval between this and the next session, and told the therapist how upset she was. Becoming very defensive, the therapist replied that she had been in practice for a number of years and that the result was not her fault at all. She then asked the client to leave. Not surprisingly, the client then sought help elsewhere.

If you should ever unfortunately find yourself in this position, try to remain calm and sympathetic. Discuss the issue with the client there and then if you feel able to and if you think the situation can be remedied fairly straightforwardly. If it is complex or if you yourself feel too upset, tell the client that you would like to discuss the issue further with colleagues (or your supervisor) in order to determine the best course of help, and give as precise an indication as you can of how long this will take and how soon you expect to get back to the client. If you think there are legal implications, make sure your notes are fully written up and consult your professional body as well as your supervisor and/or immediate colleagues. Bear in mind how you would like to be treated if you were the client.

To summarise, we can think of time-keeping and payment as a framework which helps to define the process of the therapy and the nature of the client–therapist contract. Beyond this, we believe that being aware of the implications of apparently non-therapeutic details can help us to make a consistent supportive boundary within which the client can be helped. Being professional in these aspects of our dealings with the client reinforces the professionalism of our primary therapy and models clear and effective communication, the effects of which may reach out into the client's own life and personal interactions with others.

PART

4

Taking care of the therapist: looking after yourself

Contents

15 Taking care of yourself

Taking care of yourself means, in our view, a host of things in practice. From the very beginning we have emphasised that the therapist not only transmits but in some important sense *enacts* the therapy. We began the book by inviting you to consider who you were, where you were coming from and how that affects what you have to offer the client. Now, at the other end of the book, we want you to consider yourself from another viewpoint.

If you are your own major resource, how are you going to look after yourself? It means managing your diary. It means taking rests and holidays. It means having things to think about and care about other than therapy, so that therapy remains fresh and so that you have other interests and sources of stimulus to top you up as a whole person. It means remembering how important other people (special people) are to you and making sure that they never feel they are in competition with your clients for your time and attention. It means managing all kinds of boundaries. It means saying 'no' when it might be easier to say 'yes' – and even when, sometimes, you would like to say 'yes' because there are really good reasons. It means finding ways to share the load of responsibility. It means updating your skills. It means resisting becoming solely a 'giver' – and possibly a doormat! In examining such challenges, and ways of handling them, this chapter offers some strategies for managing oneself effectively from the beginning of life as a practising therapist.

If you look back at the personal inventory you did at the beginning, you are quite likely to have identified some events and patterns of experience which led you to want to care for others. That is maybe why you have become a therapist. You may even have had more than one helping role before training as a body therapist. In your private life also you are likely to have roles which involve you in caring for others, formally or informally. As a son, daughter, partner, parent; perhaps also in voluntary roles. You are probably good at caring, and others value you for it. It has become part of your self-image, one which gives you satisfaction and sometimes pride in yourself. This is great – but it can also become a trap. It is the dilemma that helpers can find themselves in.

Put differently, what happens to your energy and your uniqueness if you devote so much to your clients that you burn out? Less dramatically, what happens to the quality of the therapy you give, to your ability to relate and respond freshly and with enthusiasm to each client, if you don't replenish your own resources?

There is only one way to say the following and that is bluntly: unless you turn the whole thing on its head and help yourself first, you will have nothing left to help others with – you could end up with 'helpers' helplessness'! Some helpers burn out and break down physically or emotionally. Some become disillusioned (if not with the therapy, then with 'the system'). Some become automata, ceasing to respond individually to their clients. Some retire early. Some die. We don't want any of these things to happen to you if we, and you, can help it.

Turn it around. What might a recipe be for an effective person-who-happens-to-be-a-therapist? The result of their effective self-management might be that they continue to enjoy their work while also enjoying life; that they have time for friends and family, and for interests that are not therapy; that they have 'time to stand and stare' (or 'waste'); that they have time and energy to grow through new interests. Just as there are therapists who die prematurely, or who burn out in other ways, there are many who live (and work) into very old age. Milton Erickson, Carl Rogers, Mother Theresa are examples. A friend who is an osteopath told us how she met a monk on an aeroplane. He was flying back to India where he was the spiritual adviser to a refugee community. During the flight he took time out to teach meditation to our friend and some of her colleagues. He was 107.

Many of the skills of self-management are quite simple. We are going to highlight some of what we have found to be the most useful ones, both because we know them to be useful in our own experience and that of our colleagues and students over the years and because they act as examples of the general principle of looking after yourself first. These skills can be grouped under the following headings:

◆ managing your time

◆ managing your physical well-being

◆ managing your personal and professional roles.

> Before you plunge in, take a few minutes to jot down what you already do under each heading. For example, under 'managing your time' you might write down 'keep a diary', 'don't work on Sundays'. Under 'managing your physical well-being', you might put 'swop treatment with colleague' or 'aerobics class' or 'giving up smoking'. For 'managing personal and professional roles', you might write 'don't treat family' or 'install answerphone'.

Some of these skills and practices may have been learned from your family experience, some from school or work. Your training course may have suggested others. We have borrowed many good ideas during our working lives from friends and colleagues. We don't believe it's necessary for anyone to reinvent the wheel! We want to share both the ideas and the reasons for them with you, to help you keep work in its place, and private and personal life in its place from the outset. We offer the ideas to you as a major way to enhance all areas of your life and to keep you as well as you hope to keep your clients!

Managing your time: dividing up your time

We use lots of metaphors to describe our relationship to time, and most of them imply that time is a form of currency. We spend it, share it, use it and waste it. In his book *The Art of Time*, Jean-Louis Servan-Schreiber said that if we substituted 'life' for 'time' in these common phrases, we would get a better sense of what we are really talking about. Reading a dull book or attending a boring meeting may be a waste of the bit of life spent there. Enjoying an evening with friends, with laughter and affection, may be an enriching way of sharing life. Many of you may have made the decision to become therapists because you felt your previous jobs were more or less a waste of your life.

The first question to ask yourself is what proportion of your time – your life – do you want to spend on work and what on other important activities. First, though, let us be clear about what we mean by 'work':

◆ Work
  - seeing clients
  - doing therapy-related administration
  - making therapy-related telephone calls
  - attending supervision sessions
  - attending workshops and further training courses
  - reading therapy-related journals.

◆ Non-work

- activities related to home, family and friends

- hobbies and sports

- community and voluntary activities/duties

- time doing nothing

- pottering.

People with 9-to-5 jobs may find it easier to make the work/non-work divide. Most helpers (e.g. social workers, therapists, teachers) have less clearly defined timetables, and often have to struggle to keep work within bounds.

One way to begin working out your own preferred ratio is to ask yourself how much you need to earn and how that equates in terms of paid hours. You may be managing a part-time job in addition to the therapy, or even, at the outset, a full-time one. However, it is important to look to the income you need as one major constraint on your decisions.

Now ask yourself how much time you want to spend working. Do the two tally with each other? For example, if you want to work 3 days a week because of family commitments, can you earn enough in those 3 days to cover your required income? How much would that mean charging each client? Would the market stand that amount? If not, where are you going to have to make the necessary adjustments?

If you have a split career at the moment, remember that travelling and 'changing hats' take both time and energy, and you may have to cut down your therapy time to allow for this.

Time available for therapy also has to include time for preparation and administration (note-taking, changing towels and laundering them). This may add up to as much as one working session's worth of time, or more, in a week. You may also have to put time aside in the evenings to return or receive phone calls; this is often easiest when people are home from work, but this eats into your private time. Work time which doesn't involve clients is the kind of time which can become a drag, for you and (perhaps even more likely) for your partner or family. Try to log how much life you spend doing these jobs, and set realistic limits for yourself which will, with discussion, be acceptable to your home-sharers. Better to say $1-1^{1}/_{2}$ hours every evening and find you can 'underspend' rather than to estimate 1 hour and regularly overspend.

Do you want to work at weekends or in the evening? Some clients will only be able to come at these times, and at the outset you may feel you need to take all the clients you can get. However, you need agreement for such encroachments into home or family time, and you may want to review this as you get busier so that you can move towards more congenial hours once you are sure you can get the work. If you decide to do administrative work in the evenings or weekends, be aware that because these focus you on work events and issues almost as much as the presence of actual clients, they will still make you and your family feel that you are working.

Organising your life: using your diary creatively

We suggest that you think of your diary as a life-management tool, not just as a record of client appointments:

◆ *Take hold of it before it takes hold of you.* Block in, weeks or even months in advance, the spaces that you intend to use for clients. That way, it's easier to say, 'I'm sorry, I haven't got any more spaces left that week', rather than sacrifice the evening you intended to catch up with the ironing/watch your favourite TV programme/catch up with friends.

◆ *Make spaces in your diary for yourself.* Give yourself equal status with your clients. Include self-maintenance (dentist, haircuts) and self-nourishment (massage, visits to the gym, lunch with a friend).

◆ *Think about how you want to feel at the end of your week* and book your appointments in accordingly. If you want lots of energy for the weekend, don't overbook yourself on Fridays.

◆ *Use the diary as a reminder.* Put in phone calls to make or bills to pay on specific days. That way you don't fill your already busy head with extra things to remember.

◆ *Think ahead and book in personal space.* Birthdays, anniversaries, school events you want to attend, days for hobbies or classes, professional development workshops. *Put them in as soon as you hear about them,* so the space is there for you if you want it. If you change your mind, you can always fill the space with work. But if you don't allocate the time in advance, you won't get it. (Imagine saying to a potential client: 'Sorry, I can't see you on Thursday because I'm taking a day off to prune the roses'.) When you get more confident, you will be able to say this kind of thing without apology, and clients will learn something useful about the value of personal time and space; but it's no good feeling you have to defend or excuse not being available.

◆ *Book time for administration.* Try leaving half an hour free at the end of a day (or starting half an hour early) or perhaps labelling one full client 'slot' as 'admin. time'. It is much easier to do the work if the time is allotted than to make a decision every time, when other pressures (or pleasures!) may incline you to leave the chores for another day.

◆ *Remember that even small amounts of time can be used fruitfully.* Better half an hour tidying, filing or reading than leaving these necessary or rejuvenating activities in the hope that a couple of hours will 'suddenly' materialise.

Managing your physical well-being

You are a body worker. You know how vital your own body is as a tool of your therapy, and your training will have taught you ways of protecting it against the special stresses of delivering your therapy day in day out. We want to broaden the view of physical maintenance a little wider and ask you to check how careful you are with yourself in a number of ways.

Diet – what you eat and drink, when you do it

When you are rushed at work, do you grab a sandwich between clients? Do you make time for a proper breakfast to sustain you through the morning? Lots of carers put their care for the clients first, at their own expense. Don't be one of them.

Exercise

Therapy is very physical work. It's also inclined to use the same muscle groups repeatedly. Remember to stretch at intervals during the working day. If possible, cultivate other forms of exercise which are fun and which also involve other muscles and movements.

Sleep

Do you get enough? Waking a lot, sleeping lightly, waking early and finding yourself thinking about work when you try to go to sleep are all warnings of stress and often of poor boundary-keeping (see Ch. 16). Take action earlier rather than later to identify causes and correct imbalances.

Physical treats and therapies

Set aside time for some physical treats for yourself. Massage, aerobics, work in the gym and swimming on a regular basis all remind you that you need care too. Some therapists swop treatments – but remember you need to make sure it feels like a treatment, not a time to chat over clients and work. If you want to do that, arrange some mutual supervision at another time.

Changing pace

Just as we can overuse muscles through repetition of particular actions, we can develop stress through repetitious pacing of our lives. If your therapy is energetic, consider activities which are slower and more fluid. If it is rhythmical and restful, what about something rapid and stimulating? Avoid becoming a one-gear person.

Managing your personal and professional roles

It is very easy for caring people to blur the boundary between personal and professional involvement. This takes various forms and is confusing for everyone concerned. We believe that being clear about which hat we are wearing is a great help to clear, effective communication. It can help us maintain all kinds of necessary boundaries. The phrase 'If you can't say no what is your yes worth?' says it very neatly. Knowing which hat you are wearing – therapist, friend or family member – at any one time allows you to be clear about which messages, duties and roles are appropriate, and which are not.

When are you a therapist? You are a therapist when you are at work (i.e. working) and when you choose to use your professional skills. You are not a therapist when you are off duty. This means that *you* will have to indicate by changes in your behaviour that you are at this moment being a private person. Sometimes the context will make it clear, but what if you meet clients in the local supermarket? Say 'Hi' rather than 'How are you?' if you want to make sure of avoiding a blow-by-blow account of their progress since their last treatment!

You do not have to be a therapist when friends or family 'invite' you to respond professionally in non-professional situations. You may need to develop some responses to their invitations. 'Give me a ring on Monday and I'll see when I have a free appointment' takes care of those whom you have decided it is permissible to treat. 'I'll just give you an off-the-cuff idea of how your problem could be approached, and the names of some colleagues who might help you, as I don't work with friends' politely maintains a boundary with others. You can make friends of clients, but don't make clients of your friends.

You have a choice. If you decide to accept the request for help, make it clear that it is an active choice, and on what terms:

> *'I can do an assessment for you, but if what you need is complex I'd prefer you to see someone else, as that keeps treatment separate from friendship.'*

Don't let yourself slip into professional discussions or 'mini-treatments' unless you want to. If you do, you will resent it and this will in turn affect the relationship you have with the other person. Naturally, you must also be clear about what payment you want for your service if you do decide to do any work, as this can be a very fruitful cause of resentment if left unclear.

You can, if you wish, trade your service with a friend or family member if it seems appropriate for something they can do for you in exchange. Sometimes this can feel really good, but be sure you discuss the nature and terms of the trade properly beforehand and that both of you feel it is fair in terms of time, effort and monetary value. It is probably better to arrange a swop within a limited time-frame, rather than having one of you give a service first with an indefinite right to 'call in' the corresponding favour: this can be harder to ask for, time-lapse may have altered the respective values and the second person may feel irrationally badgered. Unless you both have an equal and continuing need for each other's help, swopping is probably best on an occasional basis rather than as a mechanism involving sustained treatment.

Sometimes friends and family can forget, or even feel that because you are involved with them you have an obligation to help. Here as elsewhere, clear boundary-keeping and, if necessary, brief and firm explanations of its importance to both parties make for peace of mind and better relationships all round.

When clients become friends

We have already touched on various aspects of this (see Ch. 12). In our previous discussion, we were mostly concerned about spotting potential boundary issues and ensuring that no fudging occurred.

But what if you have seen the choice point and decided that friendship is what you want? A number of basic guidelines make it easier all round:

◆ *Manage the transition.* Make it clear and deliberate so that the boundary remains clear. If you and the client feel you want to become friends, agree that this is the way you feel and that you can act on it once the therapy is finished (or finish the therapy sooner so that the friendship can proceed, making other arrangements for the client to receive therapy elsewhere). In a rare number of cases, you and the client may feel fairly sure that you can continue the therapy while developing a friendship. This requires you (as the one who is responsible for the professional part of the relationship) to ask yourself and them if you think they can manage clear transitions between the two roles – can they 'change hats' and remember not only what behaviour but what knowledge belongs to which role? (Can you?) If you have any doubt, keep it simple and go for one or the other.

◆ *Talk through possible problems*. If you become friends with a client you may become part of their social circle. As their therapist, you will have a lot of information about them. Ask them how much of this you 'know' as a friend? When a client has become a friend, are they at liberty to call on your professional skills at any later point? You need to decide. If you agree that they may (on whatever basis) you will need to make it clear that in asking for professional help they will need to observe your professional boundaries, e.g. not phoning late at night (as they might with a friend) to tell you about a recurrence of their old back trouble and ask for an appointment (which is client mode). If they can't understand the need for such apparently legalistic rules, this should probably be seen as a sign that they couldn't manage the role switching easily or reliably.

◆ *Have a life outside work*, and friendship circles that don't involve clients or colleagues. Cultivate activities and people who don't know or care what it is you do for a living, but who do care about you and enjoy your company. Contacts you make through sport and exercise, hobbies or voluntary work, your children's schools (if you have them), evening classes, your neighbourhood, your friends or partner may all enlarge and enrich the social base and take pressure off your professional self. We firmly believe that someone who is only a therapist is poorer as a therapist and runs a greater and faster risk of burn-out. A close friend once said: 'Work is something I do between riding' – though in fact he was very committed to his work too. This kind of boundary-keeping takes care of the self in very important and enriching ways.

Saying no

Banks may advertise themselves as 'the one that likes to say "yes"', but we would have greater trust in a therapist who knew how and when to say 'no'.

In taking care of ourselves, saying 'no' is a front-line tool. Because most people who become therapists have a wish to offer care and support, we guess that many, if not most, people reading this (as well as many therapists who qualified years ago) will recognise that they find this difficult at times and probably remember some examples where they too readily said 'yes' only to regret it later. *If in doubt, play for time.* It is much better to say, 'Let me think that over and get back to you' than it is to say 'yes' and regret it or to say 'yes' and later have to say 'no' (and in rarer cases to have said 'no' and then changed your mind).

> Think of a recent example where you said 'yes' when someone asked something of you and have since regretted it. Ask yourself honestly why you said 'yes'. Was it to do with your view of yourself as a carer? Or to do with how you expected the speaker to feel if you refused? Or because you felt you didn't really have a choice (why)? Is it too late to retrieve the situation? If so, what can you learn from it for another time?
>
> If you frequently have trouble saying no, ask yourself if there are any patterns. Do you have trouble refusing certain kinds of requests? Or certain kinds of people? What might you need to do to modify this pattern?

In our experience, the commonest underlying problems are to do with assumptions that because we are a carer, we can't easily refuse (or shouldn't refuse) a request that comes under the label of caring (e.g. to fit in an extra appointment in a busy week); that carers must put others first (bang goes my lie-in with a good book) – in other words, that saying no is incompatible with something which we greatly value, our self-image.

As before, our solution is to take the same assumption and turn it around so that it now reads: *good carers take care of themselves in order that they have enough energy and emotional reserves to take care of their clients.* If your proposed 'no' (or the one you wish you had said) would allow you to maintain yourself better as a *holistic therapeutic tool* then it is (was/would have been) justified even according to your own criteria.

Does that feel any better?

> Spend a few moments reminding yourself how important it is to maintain and cherish yourself so that you can be a better practitioner. Now imagine being asked that same question you previously regretted saying 'yes' to. Imagine saying 'no' in a variety of ways

(with shorter and fuller explanations to take account of the circumstances and the kind of person asking). Practise till you feel comfortable. Praise yourself.

Imagine two or three similar requests and practise saying 'no' to these as well.

Imagine another situation where you felt/would feel it was right to say 'yes'. Say it. Do you feel differently about this one, having discovered that you do not have to say 'yes' all the time?

You may need to remind yourself of your *right to choose* from time to time, particularly where you are hard-pressed. It takes time to build muscle.

Learning to ask for things

Many carers find asking for things almost as difficult as saying no. Asking means we have to accept we have a *right to ask* (do carers have that right?). Many carers have cared for others long before they became professionals and may have got out of – or never developed – the habit of asking for themselves. It can feel very risky, and almost as though our professionalism was being compromised at times, to admit that we need to ask for help. We may also fear being rejected or assume that there's no point in asking because others will not have the time or will not do the job as we would do it.

Think of a recent occasion when you would have liked to ask someone for help (personally or professionally) but did not ask. What prevented you? Do you, on reflection, believe that it would have been reasonable to ask? Would you have been prepared to help them in the same way if the positions had been reversed? Think of a number of ways in which you might put your request. Did you have to convince the other person? Or yourself?

Relaxation

Any working therapist needs to develop a range of ways to relax. In our experience, the most relaxing things actually involve doing something, paradoxical though that sounds. If your work is absorbing, it's logical that something equally absorbing, but different, will help you to put work away.

For this reason, few people actually relax by flopping in front of the telly – they just give up! Turning what should be interesting or stimulating into animated wallpaper isn't relaxation. So what might be more effective?

◆ First, you need a routine for changing role and pace (see Chs 10 and 12).

◆ Then, use (if you already have them) or promise yourself to start learning (if you don't yet) some relaxation or meditative skills. Self-hypnosis, autogenics, progressive relaxation patterns, guided imagery skills and yoga all offer opportunities here. (You might consult the *Relaxation and Stress Reduction workbook* by Davis, Eshelman and McKay for a wealth of helpful options.)

◆ Plan in some nurturing for yourself on a regular basis – massage, aromatherapy or some other bodywork; visits to a health spa or club; a laze in a jacuzzi; a leisurely bath with fragrant oils.

◆ Make sure you have self-repair time for yourself *every day*, even if it is only half an hour, to use as you wish without having to account for it.

◆ Structure in to your diary regular alternative ways of being absorbed – exercise, theatre, films, meals with friends.

◆ If you like hobbies that use your hands (they need alternatives too), make regular space for them. Knitting, tapestry, sewing, bread-making, gardening all revitalise hands which spend time caring for others. Treat them to their own therapy with regular massage, nail treatments, luxurious hand creams.

◆ Give yourself the treat of a change of place. Walk or drive somewhere different. Look at detail for its own sake, not for what it needs you to do with it.

◆ Change your time-scale. Working in therapeutic slots habituates us to a certain kind of pace. Every so often it's really good to live faster, or slower, for a while just to stop being in one gear.

◆ Review your self-care programme regularly: ask yourself at the end of each day, week and month, what you have done for yourself and what difference it made. Relish the helpful, useful, wonderful, enjoyable things. Learn to adjust on a continual basis so that every day puts something back to replenish what you are continually taking out.

Supervision and support

Chapter 16 ('Being the best you can be') discusses in more detail how we can set up arrangements with other professionals which maintain and extend our skills, and which give us an important sense of connectedness in our work.

Working face-to-face with clients on an individual basis can feel lonely and at times we become very aware of the weight of decision-making and responsibility we carry on a daily basis. Regular supervision gives us the benefit of informed professional understanding and a chance to have impartial comment on our work. It means that we know we can check out difficult decisions, let go the burden of needing to be seen as confident, and learn from others' experience and different assumptions.

Putting time and love into our personal networks also repays us in a different way. Knowing there are significant others who accept us for our own unique nature and whom we value unconditionally for theirs gives us a solid foundation for all we do. Some of them have two legs: some have four (and we don't exclude tails and fins).

Key factors in self-care:

◆ Boundary management

◆ Change (is as good as...)

◆ Self-nurturing

◆ Learning to ask for things

◆ Saying 'no'

◆ Building and nurturing your support networks

16 Being the best you can be

One of the major platforms of this book has been the interconnectedness of the therapist as person and professional in their communication with the client. As a person, we are not a finite entity but, as Carl Rogers said, 'a continuous process of changingness'. So it follows that the therapist/person will be, and needs to be, continually evolving. The growth of the person enriches their therapeutic work: their therapeutic work can enrich them as a person.

There are some well-recognised means of helping professionals improve, and we want to discuss them in this chapter. We also want to explore some less obvious aids to being the best we can be.

In an earlier chapter, we talked about avoiding burn-out and suggested a number of ways of protecting and taking care of ourselves which we and other colleagues have found helpful. Many of these involved various forms of boundary-setting and boundary-keeping.

Now we want to look at maintenance from another angle. As we get further away from our initial training, we acquire more experience. We also come to rely more on that experience, interacting with it day by day, and may feel increasingly removed – not only in time – from the conceptual or methodological base of our work. For some time, the accrued experience of working with different people and different complaints (or different versions of the same complaints) will add valuably to the skills and understanding we acquired on our initial training course, so we will be becoming better therapists by this means.

But we need, even from the beginning, to be aware that excellence needs to be fostered, encouraged and nurtured, and that we have to make provision in our thinking, our time and our financial plans to do this.

Supervision

Most of the psychotherapies and different forms of social work require their practitioners to receive supervision. In many organisations, it is built into the line-management structure as a regular meeting between superiors and their subordinates. Psychotherapy professional bodies, whether their members are employed in the statutory or private sector, normally require that practitioners receive supervision for their client work, often specifying a ratio of so many hours of supervision to so many hours of client contact. Training courses often require that students in training also receive supervision as part of their learning process.

Supervision has a number of purposes. First and foremost, it protects the client, because their case will be discussed by their therapist with a practitioner who may be more experienced and who will certainly have an outside perspective on the interaction in which their therapist is involved. Where a practitioner is new to the work, supervision offers a safeguard, especially if they might be working at the edge of their understanding or skill.

Second, supervision helps the therapist. It should give any therapist moral support, help them to think their way through alternative treatments, and give them access to other case examples of a similar or different kind from which they can refine their view of this case and this client. It also allows them to become aware of issues which arise in their practice, affecting more than one client. Even when therapists are experienced, they find supervision can offer new strategies or interpretations and keep them on their toes.

Supervision is new to bodywork, although we believe it will become more widespread. Even if your training course did not require or encourage you to have supervision, we strongly urge you to arrange it for yourself.

A useful supervisor could be one of the following:

◆ someone who did the same training course and who has been in practice for a number of years

◆ someone who did a different, but well-regarded, training course and who is experienced

◆ a teacher on your training course.

You will need to meet regularly – not less than once a month, and if your practice is busy, more frequently. Normally supervision lasts for between 1 and 2 hours. You might get together with another therapist in the same field to share supervision with one supervisor: this splits the cost of the session (supervisors normally charge the same sort of fee for supervision that they would charge a client for that amount of time) and gives you the additional benefit of other cases, other issues and other ideas.

Once you become more experienced, you may want to consider a slightly different form of supervision called *peer-vision*. This involves a number of therapists (usually between two and four) with roughly equal amounts of experience getting together to discuss their work. Peer-vision needs to be clearly organised so that each member of the group feels they have had equal attention, and so that the meeting remains rigorous rather than just becoming a gossip or chat. When you are giving up potential earning time, and perhaps having to travel, you need to feel that you have gained something in terms of ideas, strategies and new perspectives as well as the enjoyment and moral support of a meeting with friendly colleagues.

A supervision session might include any of the following:

◆ discussion of individual cases either as a routine progress report or because of problems which have arisen

◆ discussion of particular techniques and their place in treatment

◆ discussion of issues arising in practice or practice management, e.g. cancellations, advertising, contracts with clinics, communications with doctors and other health professionals, patterns of reaction or response in the therapist.

Joining a professional association

Your training course is likely to have recommended a particular professional association to you. Apart from providing professional indemnity insurance for its members, an association will provide protection to both therapist and clients via a clear disciplinary procedure and, in the hopefully unlikely case of legal proceedings, legal advice and support. It will also have a published code of conduct, incorporating material on the legal responsibilities of complementary practitioners in relation to the law and the medical profession, as well as guidance on professional conduct. Make sure you read the code of conduct carefully. Some items may surprise you – e.g. the legal responsibility of complementary practitioners to inform parents that doctors, not the therapist, are responsible for matters relating to a child's health even when the parents specifically request alternative rather than allopathic treatment. (A copy of the BCMA *Code of Ethics*, covering most complementary therapies, can be obtained from the British Complementary Medical Association.)

Insurance

While it is our hope that none of you ever have a legal claim made against you, it is essential that you maintain your professional indemnity insurance, and if you are working at home check that you are covered for accidents on your premises (falling over the dog and breaking an ankle) as well as professional negligence or malpractice.

Updating knowledge and skills

When we are newly qualified, it is quite onerous enough to add fluency and experience to what we learned on our initial course! But as we gain more experience, what seemed like a ceiling of knowledge and skill begins to seem more like a plateau with other levels of expertise rising beyond it.

Updating knowledge

Professional associations often have newsletters or bulletins which update their members on developments affecting the profession.

Additionally, you may find it beneficial to join other organisations in your field – some may relate specifically to special areas of interest – or broader organisations covering a number of therapies with overlapping areas of concern.

Your training course may encourage its graduates to link up in local networks (or you might think of starting one).

You might also find out whether practitioners in your area ever meet together, even if they have received different training. This can be helpful for mutual support and network building and for mutual referrals (e.g. if you are busy or about to go on holiday).

Courses and seminars

Some associations require their members to attend a specified number of training days each year as a condition of membership. They may even arrange some for their members. Even if yours doesn't, we suggest that you make this a habit. Professional magazines, whether they are for specialist interests (e.g. *International Journal of Aromatherapy*) or more general (e.g. *Journal of Alternative and Complementary Medicine*) will usually carry adverts for day seminars or weekend workshops. Attendance is something which replenishes you – it can often be quite fun and a good opportunity to meet colleagues in your field, as well as enhancing or adding to your skills.

From the beginning, plan your finances to set aside some money for your own ongoing training and supervision. Have a separate account if you find it easier, and save a little each month. While you cannot set the cost of your initial training as a professional expense against tax, you can claim for ongoing training. So ask for and keep receipts, and get a certificate of attendance from course organisers. (This covers two purposes – it substantiates your statement to the tax inspectors and also demonstrates to your professional association that you have spent time in further training if this is required.)

Books and journals

You need to keep up to date with new developments in your field. Getting a professional journal regularly and keeping an eye on new books on your therapy, or on problems you regularly treat, help you do this.

Again, you may find it easier to budget an amount of money for this from very early on. You are then in a position to choose *which* book rather than *whether to buy* a book or not. At the beginning, you may not be earning very much, but do set aside something for yourself. Later on, when you are earning more, you can increase your budget.

Postgraduate training

Your original training body may offer further courses, either at an advanced level or of a more specialised nature. So may other training bodies in your field. As you settle into practice, you are likely to find that you become drawn towards particular areas of work (e.g. cranial osteopathy) or towards particular problems (sports injuries, hospice work). As you identify the beginnings of a specialism in yourself, think about adding formally to your expertise in this area. Further qualifications may be useful to demonstrate this additional expertise to clients or to employers, and will usefully go on your CV. Would you rather see a practitioner with one set of qualifications and '15 years in practice' on their card, or one with several sets of qualifications? Fifteen years in practice, as one cynic pointed out, may mean year 1's work repeated 15 times! Of course, it may also mean 15 years of evolving and developing skill. We are inclined to believe that good practitioners find from time to time that they have reached a plateau, and begin to look for a new stimulus and new understanding to stretch themselves and add to their work.

Skills audit

A useful self-help mechanism is to set aside time at a regular interval (your birthday? 31st December? every quarter day?) to reflect on yourself as a practitioner. Ask yourself what you are good at, what you feel you could improve, where you feel you are heading professionally, what help or additional impetus you need and where you will find it. Make a brief note of your 'findings' and decisions. As each successive audit time comes around, look back at what you wrote last time and review progress honestly – and also charitably!

You could also ask your supervisor to help you carry out this audit by helping you to reflect, examine and clarify your thinking and your practice. (For further information on the process of supervision, you could consult Hawkins & Shohett's useful conceptual book, *Supervision in the Helping Professions*, or Gaie Huston's practical and user-friendly *Supervision*, available from the Rochester Foundation.)

Because we are people who happen to be therapists, the audit needs to include not just an assessment of our professional work and targets for future development, but a more personal evaluation of our own experiences outside work and how these have affected and enriched us as a whole. Taking time to reflect on what has happened in our lives since our last audit often highlights important learnings which interconnect our personal and professional selves.

Acquiring new, linked skills

Many therapists find that as they gain experience they feel that they could usefully add another related skill to their own. Some even feel this during their initial training. Aromatherapists may be drawn towards reflexology or kineseology, and massage therapists towards energy work. Or you may become aware that some clients' problems have a dietary or psychological component, and wonder about additional training in those therapies as an adjunct to your primary therapy. Having a range of knowledge can enrich you and your practice, but remember also that clients will probably come looking for one therapy and that you will still need a clear focus (or at most two) for your work.

Learning something new can be refreshing and this meets another need which we have as professionals: to be stretched and stimulated and to take in as well as to give out. From this viewpoint, learning homoeopathy may benefit you even if you never intend to work as a homoeopath!

One word of caution. Being a learner reminds us of what we don't know, and it is therefore very important, if we are involved in substantial further training, to reinforce our confidence at regular intervals so that we are not unintentionally undermining our own base. In our experience, the first effect of a workshop or training event is actually *de-skilling*, because it makes us bring into conscious focus all those processes we have been operating with unconscious competence (rather like the effect of driving a different make of car, we have to think afresh about the gearing, the width, the effectiveness of the brakes). Usually it takes a little time for the new skill or knowledge to become integrated into our automatic, unconsciously managed repertoire. It can be helpful to remember this when attending training and to give ourselves permission *not* to try to use the new learning immediately in our practice, but to allow it time to drift in naturally.

Being aware of the 'I need more information' trap

Having high standards, you will be aware that there is always more to know about your therapy. Talking with colleagues, including your supervisor, attending workshops, reading professional journals, all remind you of what lies at the edges of your own body of knowledge and skill. It can be easy for the conscientious person to feel obliged to keep adding, searching and topping up. While we have argued that refreshing oneself and adding to one's bag of tools are important, it is also important to keep reminding ourselves of *what we can already do* and *what we do well*. The psychiatrist Donald Winnicott drew attention to this over-commitment to excellence, and its debilitating effects, when he coined the phrase 'the good enough parent'. We believe we need to have in mind the notion of being a 'good enough therapist' – although this includes being aware of the limits of our skill and knowledge, it also involves an honest awareness of what we are good at, what is special in how we relate to our clients and what we offer them.

Winnicott argued that parents shouldn't berate themselves for not living up to their ideals of parenting, but recognise that children are charitable and resilient, and can flourish even if mistakes are made, providing the parents are honest, value them and take them seriously. The American psychotherapist, Carl Rogers, identified three key elements in good therapists: genuineness, empathy and non-possessive warmth. It is our experience that therapists of all disciplines and persuasions help many varieties of client when they start from this kind of base.

So we end the book as we began – with the belief that the best you can offer your clients as a means of helping them with their difficulties is a living and continuously evolving resource: what you know, what you can do and also what you are.

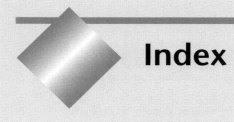

Index